CAMBRIDGE LIBRARY COLLECTION

Books of enduring scholarly value

History of Medicine

It is sobering to realise that as recently as the year in which On the Origin of Species was published, learned opinion was that diseases such as typhus and cholera were spread by a 'miasma', and suggestions that doctors should wash their hands before examining patients were greeted with mockery by the profession. The Cambridge Library Collection reissues milestone publications in the history of Western medicine as well as studies of other medical traditions. Its coverage ranges from Galen on anatomical procedures to Florence Nightingale's common-sense advice to nurses, and includes early research into genetics and mental health, colonial reports on tropical diseases, documents on public health and military medicine, and publications on spa culture and medicinal plants.

The Influence of Climate in the Prevention and Cure of Chronic Diseases

Published in 1829, this important work raised awareness of a poorly understood topic, running to a third edition by 1841. Sir James Clark (1788–1870) had trained as a surgeon in Edinburgh and gained experience in the Royal Navy during the Napoleonic Wars. During subsequent European travels, he studied the effects of climate on disease, particularly tuberculosis, and this publication represents an expanded version of his *Medical Notes on Climate, Diseases, Hospitals, and Medical Schools in France, Italy, and Switzerland* (1820), which is also reissued in this series. A licentiate of the Royal College of Physicians from 1826, and elected to the Royal Society in 1832, Clark became a trusted physician and friend to Queen Victoria and Prince Albert. Also reissued in the Cambridge Library Collection are his *Treatise on Pulmonary Consumption* (1835) and *Memoir of John Conolly* (1869).

T0188060

Cambridge University Press has long been a pioneer in the reissuing of out-of-print titles from its own backlist, producing digital reprints of books that are still sought after by scholars and students but could not be reprinted economically using traditional technology. The Cambridge Library Collection extends this activity to a wider range of books which are still of importance to researchers and professionals, either for the source material they contain, or as landmarks in the history of their academic discipline.

Drawing from the world-renowned collections in the Cambridge University Library and other partner libraries, and guided by the advice of experts in each subject area, Cambridge University Press is using state-of-the-art scanning machines in its own Printing House to capture the content of each book selected for inclusion. The files are processed to give a consistently clear, crisp image, and the books finished to the high quality standard for which the Press is recognised around the world. The latest print-on-demand technology ensures that the books will remain available indefinitely, and that orders for single or multiple copies can quickly be supplied.

The Cambridge Library Collection brings back to life books of enduring scholarly value (including out-of-copyright works originally issued by other publishers) across a wide range of disciplines in the humanities and social sciences and in science and technology.

The Influence of Climate in the Prevention and Cure of Chronic Diseases

JAMES CLARK

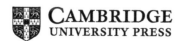

CAMBRIDGE
UNIVERSITY PRESS

CAMBRIDGE
UNIVERSITY PRESS

University Printing House, Cambridge, CB2 8BS, United Kingdom

Published in the United States of America by Cambridge University Press, New York

Cambridge University Press is part of the University of Cambridge.

It furthers the University's mission by disseminating knowledge in the pursuit of education, learning and research at the highest international levels of excellence.

www.cambridge.org
Information on this title: www.cambridge.org/9781108062312

© in this compilation Cambridge University Press 2013

This edition first published 1829
This digitally printed version 2013

ISBN 978-1-108-06231-2 Paperback

THE

INFLUENCE OF CLIMATE

IN THE

PREVENTION AND CURE

OF

CHRONIC DISEASES,

MORE PARTICULARLY OF

THE CHEST AND DIGESTIVE ORGANS:

COMPRISING

AN ACCOUNT OF THE PRINCIPAL PLACES

RESORTED TO BY INVALIDS IN

ENGLAND AND THE SOUTH OF EUROPE ;

A COMPARATIVE ESTIMATE OF THEIR

RESPECTIVE MERITS IN PARTICULAR DISEASES ;

AND

GENERAL DIRECTIONS FOR INVALIDS

WHILE TRAVELLING AND RESIDING ABROAD.

———

𝖂𝖎𝖙𝖍 𝖆𝖓 𝕬𝖕𝖕𝖊𝖓𝖉𝖎𝖝, 𝖈𝖔𝖓𝖙𝖆𝖎𝖓𝖎𝖓𝖌 𝖆 𝕾𝖊𝖗𝖎𝖊𝖘 𝖔𝖋 𝕿𝖆𝖇𝖑𝖊𝖘 𝖔𝖓 𝕮𝖑𝖎𝖒𝖆𝖙𝖊.

———

BY JAMES CLARK, M. D.

MEMBER OF THE ROYAL COLLEGE OF PHYSICIANS OF LONDON ;

CORRESPONDING MEMBER OF THE ROYAL MEDICAL SOCIETY OF MARSEILLES, OF THE
MEDICO-CHIRURGICAL SOCIETY OF NAPLES, OF THE MEDICAL AND PHYSICAL SOCIETY
OF FLORENCE, OF THE ACADEMY OF SCIENCES OF SIENNA, &c. &c.

———

LONDON:

THOMAS AND GEORGE UNDERWOOD,

32, FLEET STREET.

———

MDCCCXXIX.

TO

JOHN FORBES, M.D. F.R.S.

SENIOR PHYSICIAN OF THE CHICHESTER INFIRMARY,

AS A TRIBUTE JUSTLY DUE

TO HIS

VIRTUES, TALENTS, AND ACQUIREMENTS,

AND

TO HIS ZEAL IN

THE ADVANCEMENT OF MEDICAL SCIENCE:

AND AS

THE MEMORIAL OF A FRIENDSHIP

THAT HAS BEEN THE

SOURCE OF MUCH HAPPINESS AND MANY BENEFITS:

This Work is Inscribed

BY HIS FAITHFUL AND ATTACHED FRIEND,

THE AUTHOR.

PREFACE.

It is nearly nine years since I published a small volume of " Notes " on the Climate and Medical Institutions of France and Italy. This met with a very favourable reception ; more, I believe, from the want of such a work, than from any merit it possessed. Since that time I have had ample opportunities of observing the nature of the climate of the south of Europe, and its effects on disease : and during the three years which have elapsed since my return from the Continent, I have endeavoured to make myself acquainted with the milder parts of England, with the view of ascertaining their respective merits, and of comparing them with the climates of the south. The present work may, therefore, be considered as exhibiting the result of much more extended observation and experience than its predecessor.

But although I have endeavoured to take a more comprehensive and philosophical view of my subject, I wish this work still to be regarded as an Essay, which future and yet more extensive observation can only perfect. If, however, it shall be found that I have investigated the subject faithfully and closely, as far as I have gone, and if the results of my researches, and my experience, now recorded, shall prove useful to future inquirers, and serve as a guide to my medical brethren in the application of climate to the prevention and cure of disease, I trust I may be considered as having accomplished all that could be reasonably expected of me, in an inquiry of such extent and difficulty.

The following work is divided into two parts. In the FIRST, I have endeavoured to determine the general physical characters of the milder climates of the South of Europe and of England,—to point out the manner in which the climate of different

places resorted to by invalids is modified
by local circumstances; and to compare
these places relatively to their influence on
disease.

This part is illustrated by a series of
meteorological tables (which will be found
in the Appendix) more comprehensive and
perfect, I believe, than have before been
published; and for the construction of
which I am indebted to the kindness of
my friend Dr. Todd.

In the SECOND PART, I have given some
account of the principal diseases which are
benefited by a mild climate. This I found
to be unavoidable; it being impossible,
otherwise, to give precise directions for the
application of particular climates to the cure
of particular diseases,—and much more so
to their varieties and complications.

In my endeavours to distinguish the characters of some of these diseases in relation
to the effects of climate upon them, it may
appear that I have been unnecessarily
minute; but I have only made such dis-

tinctions as my experience warranted ; and
I have made them, because I feel satisfied
that without strict attention to distinctions
of this kind, climate can never be successfully applied as a remedial agent.

In treating of two diseases (or rather
classes of disease) I have gone more into
detail than the nature of my work may,
at first sight, appear to require ; but the
great importance of these affections, their
extreme frequency in this country, and the
close relation in which they stand to climate,
considered as a remedy, appeared to me to
claim for them all the consideration which
I have bestowed upon them.

The diseases to which I allude are Consumption, and Disorders of the Digestive
Organs. Under this last title, I comprehend
the various affections designated by the
terms " Indigestion," " Bilious Complaints,"
&c. In the article on Consumption, I have
endeavoured to show that the disordered
states of the stomach are intimately connected with the origin of diseases of the chest,
and with tuberculous affections generally. On

this account alone disorders of the digestive organs would claim particular notice in a work of this kind; but on their own account they are no less entitled to attention, seeing the amount of suffering and of evil which they produce, and the great benefit which I have shown may be derived from change of air and of climate in the treatment of them.

With respect to the subject of Consumption, it will probably be considered the most legitimate of any, in a work treating of the effects of climate. On this occasion, I have directed my inquiries chiefly to the causes and origin of this fatal disease, with the view of establishing rules for its prevention; being well satisfied that it is only by a knowledge of the causes which lead to it, and by directing our efforts to counteract them, that we shall be able to diminish the ravages of Consumption. On this most important inquiry, therefore, I have entered as fully as the nature of my work would admit, and have endeavoured, to the best of my abilities, to fill up the blark which has been left in the natural

history of Consumption,—that, namely, between a state of health, and of established
and sensible disease of the lungs.

I feel convinced that by adopting such
a system of management, from early infancy,
as I have laid down in the following pages,
a great improvement might be effected in
the general health of many among the higher
and middle classes of society in this country.
The children of delicate, and even of diseased parents, might, by proper care, be
reared so as to overcome, in a large proportion of cases, their hereditary disposition
to disease. The ultimate effect of this in
diminishing the vast and increasing extent
of hereditary diseases, need not be pointed
out.

Instructions respecting the necessary pre-
paration of invalids for a change of climate,—
for their guidance during the journey, and
during their residence abroad, will be found
as minutely laid down as the nature of the
subject would admit. During my residence
on the Continent, I found these matters
greatly neglected. They are, however, of

the very first consequence to invalids, as, without attention to them, the best climate will be productive of little benefit.

It was originally my intention to have added a third part, giving some account of the principal mineral waters of the Continent; but I found, on arranging my materials on this subject, that I could not have condensed them sufficiently for this purpose, without greatly diminishing their value. I have therefore resolved to lay them before the public in a separate volume; and have satisfied myself, on the present occasion, with merely indicating the mineral waters most suitable to the different diseases treated of. This class of remedies will be found to co-operate powerfully with a mild climate in the removal of many chronic disorders.

This is the proper place to notice the kind and liberal assistance which I have received from many friends, while engaged in collecting materials for this work. To Drs. Heineken and Renton of Madeira, Dr. Skirving of Nice, Dr. Peebles of Rome, and Dr. Playfair of Florence, I am indebted

for much valuable information. By the
assistance chiefly of the two first named
gentlemen, I have been enabled to give
more precise information respecting the
climate of Madeira, and its influence on
disease, than has, I believe, been previously
laid before the public. From Dr. Forbes of
Chichester, Dr. Lempriere of Newport, and
Dr. Down of Southampton, I have received
much information respecting several of the
English climates. But the gentleman to
whom I am indebted above all others, is my
esteemed friend Dr. Todd of Brighton, who
has, with one or two exceptions, resided for
some time at all the places on the Continent
noticed in the following pages, and who has
unreservedly communicated to me the result
of his observations and extensive experience;
so that there is scarcely an article in the
work which has not been improved by his
suggestions. I also avail myself of the present
occasion, with much pleasure, to acknowledge
the information which I liberally received
from my continental brethren. To my
valued friends, Professor De Matthæis of
Rome, Dr. Lanza of Naples, Dr. Mojon of
Genoa, and Professor Grotanelli of Sienna,

I am more particularly indebted in this way. Indeed, the friendly and liberal intercourse which I enjoyed, while on the Continent, with my professional brethren, is one of the circumstances connected with my residence abroad, the retrospect of which affords me the greatest satisfaction. I can assure such of the profession of this country as may visit the Continent, that they will very generally experience there the greatest facility in prosecuting their professional researches; and, I take leave to add, that, if they carry with them minds free from prejudice, and a sufficient degree of practical knowledge to enable them to profit by what they observe, they will not fail to improve themselves.

I hope it will be found that I have succeeded in throwing some light on the obscure subject of the influence of climate on human health, and on the application of it to the treatment of disease. I would also hope, from the minute manner in which I have described the characters of the different climates frequented by invalids, and the care with which I have indicated the nature of the diseases benefited by them, that I

have gone far to correct many of the erroneous opinions which have hitherto existed
on these subjects. However this may be,
I do at least anticipate this good effect
from my labours — that, for the future,
those patients only will be sent abroad whose
cases afford a reasonable prospect of benefit
from such a measure ; and, that the practice
of hurrying out of their own country a class
of invalids, whose sufferings can only be
thereby increased, and their lives shortened,
will no longer be sanctioned, but that such
persons may be allowed, henceforth, to die
in peace in the bosom of their own families.

As I anticipated that the following work
would be perused by many persons not of
the profession, but who are yet deeply
interested in the subject of climate, in
relation to its effects on disease, I have
endeavoured to express myself in as plain
language as possible ; and I trust I have
succeeded in making myself intelligible to
the generality of readers, without at all
diminishing the utility of my book to the
members of my own profession. It has been
my wish to lay before the public such a work

as might serve at once as a manual to the physician in selecting a proper climate for his patient, and a guide to the latter while no longer under the direction of his medical adviser. It is only those who have resided abroad, and have mixed much with that numerous class of our countrymen who travel for health, that can know how very much such a publication is wanted; and I may perhaps be permitted to add, at the same time, that it is only those who have attempted to compose such a work that can be aware of the difficulties of the task.

George-Street, Hanover-Square,
May 22, 1829.

CONTENTS.

PART THE FIRST.

ON CLIMATE.

MADEIRA.

PART THE SECOND.

———

CONSUMPTION.

CHRONIC RHEUMATISM.

GENERAL DELICACY OF CONSTITUTION IN CHILDHOOD AND YOUTH.

PREMATURE DECAY AT A MORE ADVANCED PERIOD OF LIFE.

DISORDERED HEALTH FROM HOT CLIMATES.

APPENDIX.

—

TABLES ON CLIMATE, &c.

INFLUENCE OF CLIMATE

ON

CHRONIC DISEASES,

&c. &c.

Plurimi morbi, nullis aliis remediis domandi, tempestate vel cœlo mutato sponte evanescunt, aut levantur : Et omnes medici, tam veteres quam recentiores, in hoc consentiunt, cœli mutationem multum esse auxilii in variis morbis, vix aliter medendis.—GREGORY.

PART THE FIRST.

ON CLIMATE.

INTRODUCTORY REMARKS.

ALTHOUGH the power of different climates to produce as well as to alleviate and cure diseases, is well established as a matter of fact, yet, perhaps, there is nothing in general science more unsatisfactory than the manner in which we are able to explain this influence; and certainly there is nothing in physic more difficult than to direct successfully its application. Much of this arises from the natural difficulties of the subject, but much also from our neglect of careful observation. And yet when it is recollected that the problem of physical climate still remains unsolved by natural philosophers, it need not be matter of surprize that the physician should find it no easy matter, nay almost impossible, to give a satisfactory explanation, when the subject becomes complicated by the addition of such elements as organic life, health and disease, with all the intricacy and complexity of their combinations. " When we study the organic life of plants and animals," says Humboldt, " we must examine all the stimuli or external agents which modify their vital actions. The ratios of the mean temperatures of the months are not sufficient to characterize the climate. Its influence combines the simultaneous action of all physical causes; and it depends on heat, humidity, light, the electrical tension of vapours, and the variable pressure of the atmosphere. In making known the empirical laws of the distribution of heat over the globe, as deducible from the thermometrical variations of the air, we are far from considering these laws as the only ones necessary to resolve all the problems of climate. Most of the phenomena of nature present two distinct points, one which may be subjected to exact calculation, and another which cannot be reached but through the medium of induction and analogy."* No one can be more sensible of the truth of these remarks than myself; and, indeed, I have cited them to show, that,

* On Isothermal lines.

although the utmost diligence has been used to
determine the physical characters of the different
climates, more especially as regards temperature,
(unquestionably the principal element of climate,)
such is the imperfect state of our knowledge on
this subject, that in this, as well as in my endeavours to trace the relations between different
climates and the human body in health and
disease, I have been obliged to content myself, in
a great measure, with simply detailing the un-
explained results of experience. It will be my
endeavour, however, in the following pages to
state, as far as the data with which I have been
able to furnish myself enable me—first, the physical characters of the different climates; secondly,
the experience of the effects of these; and finally,
the characteristic, or, if I may so express myself,
the medicinal qualities of each particular climate,
as deduced from the combined results of the two
preceding sources of information.

The influence of climate in the prevention and
cure of diseases is, for many reasons, a subject
of peculiar interest to the inhabitants of this
country. To the inclemency of our seasons we
are justified in attributing some of our most fatal
diseases; and many others, of great frequency,
if they do not derive their origin immediately from
our climate, are at least greatly aggravated by it.
Among this number may be ranked pulmonary
consumption, and some other fatal diseases of the

chest ; scrofulous affections ; rheumatism ; disorders of the digestive organs ; hypochondriasis,
and a numerous train of nervous disorders, &c.
For the prevention of some, and the cure of
others of these diseases, a temporary residence
in a milder climate is the best, often the only
effectual remedy we possess.

Change of climate and change of air have
been considered by physicians as remedial agents
of great efficacy from a very early period ; and
the correctness of the opinion is supported both
by reason and experience. It is reasonable, for
example, to believe, that a change of residence
from a crowded city to the country, or from a
cold exposed part of the country to a warmer
and more sheltered one, or from a confined, humid
valley, to a dry elevated situation, or the reverse,
would produce very sensible effects on the living
body ; and we find by daily experience that such
is the case. The marked improvement of the
general health, effected by a change from a great
city to the country, even for a short period, is
matter of daily remark ; and the suspension, or
even cure, of various diseases by a removal from
one part of the country to another, is an occurrence that must have come within the observation
of every one. It may suffice to mention here, in
reference to this fact, intermittent fevers, asthma,
catarrhal affections, hooping cough, dyspepsia,
hypochondriasis, and certain nervous disorders.

All these diseases are frequently suspended, and often entirely cured, by simple change of situation, after they had long resisted medical treatment; or they are found to yield, under the influence of such a change, to remedies that previously made little or no impression upon them.

If such marked results are produced by a change of so limited an extent as has just been noticed, it is surely reasonable to expect that a complete change of climate, together with the circumstances necessarily connected with this, should produce still more important results in ameliorating the general health, and in preventing and curing diseases: and in this expectation we are again borne out by experience.

Unfortunately, however, for the character of this remedy, it has too often been resorted to either as a last resource, or forlorn hope, in cases which were almost hopeless; or it has been mis-applied in cases wherein it might have been of essential service. Patients, who really might have derived much benefit from climate, have been too often sent abroad without proper directions re-specting the situation most suited to their com-plaints, and altogether uninstructed respecting various circumstances, a due attention to which could alone render the best selected climate bene-ficial to them.

Under such circumstances, it need not excite

our surprise, that success has not more generally
attended the practice of sending invalids abroad;
nor even, that the result should have been such
as to bring the remedy into discredit. The fault,
however, is to be sought for, not in the remedy,
but in the manner in which it has been prescribed.
My own experience, the result of extensive observation, satisfies me, that, for the prevention
and cure of a numerous class of chronic diseases,
we possess in change of climate, and even in the
more limited measure of change of air in the
same climate, one of our most powerful remedial
agents; and one, too, for which, in many cases,
we have no adequate substitute.

On the continent, the beneficial effects of
change of air are duly estimated; and the inhabitants of this country, and more especially of
this metropolis, are now becoming fully sensible
of its value. The vast increase in the size of our
watering places, of late years, and the deserted
state of London during several months, are sufficient proofs, not to mention others, of the
increasing conviction among the public in general,
that, for the preservation of health, it is necessary,
from time to time, to change the relaxing, I may
say deteriorating air of London, for the more
pure and invigorating air of the country. This,
indeed, is the best, if not the only remedy, for
that terrible malady which preys upon the vitals,

and stamps its hues upon the countenance of almost every permanent resident in this great city, and which may be justly termed the *Cachexia Londinensis*. When the extent of benefits which may be derived from this remedy, both on the physical and moral constitution, is duly estimated, no person whose circumstances permit him to avail himself of it, will fail to do so.

But even in cases of this kind, the remedy, simple as it appears, must not be applied indiscriminately and without consideration. In that numerous class of persons, indeed, who are merely suffering from a residence in the city, without any decided disease, the simple change to the country may be all that is requisite to restore their health, and it is of less consequence to what part of the country they go. But the case is very different with the real invalid, whose sufferings are chiefly referable to some particular disease. To him, the selection of his temporary residence is not a matter of indifference. For one individual of this kind, an elevated situation and a dry bracing air, will be most proper; a sheltered residence, with a milder air, will be suitable to another; while the sea-side may be the situation indicated for a third. In like manner is it with the more important measure of change of climate. In the case of the valetudinarian, in whom the feelings and functions of health are merely deteriorated by too close application to business, &c., and to whom relaxation of mind is as requisite as change of climate, we may permit the patient to choose the situation which is most agreeable to himself. But the great difference which exists in the physical characters of the climates of the places frequented by invalids in the South of Europe, and even in the southern parts of our own island, renders the selection of a winter residence for the invalid suffering under actual disease, a matter of vital importance.

This is a subject which has, unfortunately, been little attended to ; and the neglect of it has, I believe, arisen, in a great measure, from the opinion which has generally prevailed in this country, that climate is chiefly useful in consumptive diseases. Such an opinion could only have originated in a very limited acquaintance with the influence of climate on disease ; and, indeed, it is so far from being a correct view of the matter, that, were the character of this remedy to be estimated by its effects on consumption, when fully formed, it would be justly valued at a very low rate. In dyspepsia, and disorders of the digestive organs generally, and in the nervous affections and distressing mental feelings which so often accompany these ; in hypochondriasis, in asthma, in bronchial diseases, in scrofula, and in rheumatism, the beneficial effects of climate are often far more strongly evinced than they are in consumption. Likewise, in cases of general delicacy of constitution and derangement of the system, in childhood and in youth, which cannot be classed strictly under any of these diseases; and in that disordered state of the general health which so often occurs at a certain period of more advanced life, when the powers of the constitution, both mental and bodily, are apt to fail, and the system to lapse into a state of premature decay, change of climate becomes a most powerful remedy.

The mere *act of travelling* over a considerable extent of country is itself a remedy of great value, and, when judiciously conducted, will materially assist the beneficial effects of climate. A journey may indeed be regarded as a continuous and rapid change of climate, as well as of scene; and constitutes a remedy of unequalled power in some of those morbid states of the system in which the mind suffers as well as the body. The continued change of air seems to do that for the corporeal part, which the constant succession of new scenes and objects does for the mind. In chronic irritation of the mucous surfaces of the pulmonary and digestive organs, especially when complicated with a morbidly sensitive state of the nervous system, in hypochondriasis, &c., travelling will often effect more than any other remedy with which I am acquainted.

But neither travelling nor change of climate, nor the combined influence of both, will produce much permanent benefit unless directed with due regard to the nature of the case, and aided by proper regimen. And here I beg to caution the invalid, who goes abroad for the recovery of his health, not to expect too much from the mere change of climate. The air, or climate, is often regarded by patients as possessing some specific power by virtue of which it directly cures the disease. This is a very erroneous view of the matter, and not unfrequently proves the bane of the invalid, by leading him, in the fulness of his confidence in climate, to neglect other circumstances, an attention to which may be as essential to his recovery as even that in which all his hopes are placed.

A residence in a mild climate will, no doubt, often do much, but it will seldom do all that is necessary. Among other advantages, for example, it will enable the invalid to be much in the open air during a part of the year when he would be either confined to the house in this country, or exposed to an atmosphere more likely to increase than mitigate his complaints. The frequent exercise thus enjoyed in a temperate atmosphere, while it improves the general health, will relieve the affected organs, by promoting and maintaining a more free and regular circulation

in the surface and extremities. And while the
bodily health is thus improved, the mind very
generally comes in for its share of the benefit.
The new scenes and the objects of interest, with
which the South of Europe, more especially Italy,
abounds, exert a direct and beneficial influence on
the mental constitution; and this influence will,
in many cases, be greatly assisted, in an indirect
manner, by the necessary subtraction of the invalid
from many causes of care and anxiety, in other
words, from many sources of disease, to which he
would have been exposed at home.

These are some of the more obvious advantages
which the invalid may expect to derive from a
residence in a foreign climate; and they are assuredly great advantages: but if he would reap
the full measure of good which his new position
places within his reach, he must trust more to
himself and to his own conduct, than to the simple
influence of climate, however genial. He must
adhere strictly to such a mode of living as his case
requires; and he must exercise both courage and
patience in prosecuting this to a successful issue.

In the body of the work I shall have many
opportunities of pointing out how genially yet
powerfully the various circumstances connected
with change of climate operate in the renovation
of constitutions broken down by the long continuance of chronic diseases. I shall also have

occasion to expose, at greater length, the various ways in which such great and beneficial effects are produced. At present, however, I wish rather to impress the mind of the invalid with the danger of trusting too much to climate. Here, as in every other department of the healing art, we must be guided by experience ; and must rest satisfied with the amount of power which medicine concedes to us. The charlatan may boast of a specific remedy for many or for all diseases ; the man of science knows that there exists hardly a single remedy which can warrant such a boast ; and that it is only by acting on and through the numerous and compli- cated functions of the living body, (often slowly,) in various ways and by various means, and by care- fully adapting our agents to the circumstances of each particular case, that we can check or remove the disorders of the animal system, more especially chronic affections which have long existed. Let it not then be imagined that change of climate, how- ever powerful as a remedy, can be considered, in its mode of action, as totally different from other remedies, or as justifying, either on the part of the physician or patient, the neglect of those pre- cautions which are requisite to ensure the proper action of all our therapeutical means. Had I not considered this remedy as of the greatest value, and deserving the utmost attention of medical men in the cases of those who have the means of making a trial of it, I never should have undertaken the present work; but I should feel that I were at once compromising the dignity and honour of my profession, and acting in direct opposition to the lessons of experience, if I admitted, for a moment, that it is one possessing *specific* powers, and which may be indiscriminately applied without regard to the general and fundamental principles of medical science. In this case, as in that of every other therapeutical agent, I conscientiously and cordially subscribe to the confession of faith of the great Boerhaave,—" Nullum ego cognosco remedium nisi quod tempestivo usu fiat tale."

In taking a general survey of the climates of the different places resorted to by invalids for the amelioration of their health, we shall find that some bear a close resemblance to each other in certain general features, whilst others are in almost every respect diametrically opposite. Thus, we find that the South-West of England (with the exception of the extreme western point of the peninsula of Cornwall, which has a climate peculiar to itself) resembles very closely the South-West of France; that the South-East of France is opposed in every respect to the South-West of France; that the climate of Italy differs from both; that the climate of Nice partakes of the qualities of the Italian as well as of that of Pro-

vence ; and that Madeira, or the climate of the
Eastern Atlantic, can be classed with neither of
the foregoing.

These general distinctions lead to a natural
grouping, or classification, of climates, which will
materially assist us in our undertaking. And we
shall find, moreover, that each of these divisions
has some leading quality in the nature of its
climate, which distinguishes it from the others,
and which, in a medical point of view, is very
important.

————

ENGLAND.

———

BEFORE travelling beyond sea in search of a climate that may prove beneficial to his disease, the invalid will naturally inquire what resources, in this respect, the limits of our own Island afford. And I am inclined to believe that England possesses advantages which have not been made so fully available in this way, as they might have been; and that many invalids, for want of discrimination in applying the proper climates to the diseases to which they are most suited, have gone abroad in search of that which they might have found almost at their own doors.

LONDON.

In taking our departure from London, as, for obvious reasons, the most important point in our survey, it is necessary to observe, in the outset, how much of the peculiarities of its present climate it owes to artificial circumstances. Under this

head we must take into account the effects of a
crowded assemblage of so many living beings, and
the multifarious processes ministering to their
existence; the countless operations of art; the
influence of buildings, &c., in augmenting and
diffusing warmth, by reflection, by radiation, and
in other ways. Besides these more direct effects,
the more indirect influence of perfect draining and
of paving, in contributing to maintain a dry state
of the soil and of the atmosphere, ought not to
be forgotten.

The above-mentioned circumstances all tend,
some in a greater, others in a less degree, to the
creation of a peculiar climate in London. As
regards temperature, we have their influence very
accurately shown; but the subject becomes more
difficult when we would discover the other elements which constitute the complex problem of
climate.

The mean annual temperature of London is
50° 39, being one and a half degree above that
of the environs, with the exception, perhaps, of
the warmer parts of Brompton and Chelsea, which
are acknowledged to be peculiarly sheltered.*

This difference of temperature between the
metropolis and surrounding country, as the physician ought to know, is very unequally distributed

* The temperature of the environs is calculated from
Howard's observations made at *Plaistow*, *Stratford* and *Tot-
tenham-Green*.

throughout the year, and throughout the day. The excess of the city temperature arrives at its maximum in January, at which time it exceeds that of the environs by three degrees; but the difference throughout the whole of the winter, is less than it is in the summer. In the spring months, the temperature of the environs becomes nearly equal to that of London, and in the month of May it rather exceeds it. The excess of the city temperature is greatest in the months of January, September, November, and August; and the relative degree of excess is in the order stated. That accurate observer, Howard, further shows, that this excess of temperature of the city " belongs, in strictness, to the *nights;* which average three degrees and seven-tenths warmer than in the country; while the heat of the day, owing, without doubt, to the interruption of a portion of the solar rays by a constant veil of smoke, falls, on a mean of years, about a third of a degree short of that on the plain."* As was also to have been expected, the temperature of London does not show so extensive a range between its extremes, either during the year, the month, or the day, as the temperature of its environs; and the amount of variation between the successive days, which shows the steadiness of temperature, is also considerably less in the

* Climate of London, Vol. ii., p. 289.

former than in the latter. It will be the duty of
the physician to weigh against these advantages
in point of temperature, which London possesses,
countervailing ones of a different character ; and
to decide how far some gain in warmth, (more
particularly in the night,) in steadiness of temperature, and in a greater degree of dryness and
stillness, is counterbalanced by a diminution of
the purity of the atmosphere, and other qualities.
of climate.

I shall not at present enter more fully upon the
consideration of the Climate of London : its
peculiarities will be made more apparent in the
sequel, by the frequent comparisons which we
shall have occasion to make between it and the
other climates, which we purpose to describe.

SOUTH COAST OF ENGLAND.*

Leaving London, we naturally first turn our
view in search of a milder climate, to the *Southern*

* The mild region of England admits of being divided into
four districts, or groupes of Climate : That of the *South Coast*,
comprehending the tract of coast between Hastings and Port-
land Island ; the *South-West Coast*, from the latter point to
Cornwall ; the district of the *Land's-End ;* the *Western Groupe*,
comprehending the places along the borders of the Bristol
channel and æstuary of the Severn. We shall find that each of
these regions has some peculiar features in its climate which
characterize it, and distinguish it from the others, both as regards
its physical and medical qualities.

Coast of our island. Various places along this extensive and populous coast, are more or less frequented by invalids, who migrate from the northern and interior parts of the island in search of milder seasons; but here, as elsewhere, we have to regret that more registers of the weather have not been kept. For want of more general data, our observations can only apply correctly to *Hastings, Brighton, Chichester, Gosport, South-ampton* and the *Isle of Wight*.

Were we to rest contented with the result of the mean annual temperature, we should find that there was very little difference between that of the Southern Coast and of London. But when we descend from generalities to particulars, we observe that there does exist a considerable differ-ence in their temperature, arising from the manner of its distribution. It is because the climate of London and the interior of the island, com-pensates by the excess of heat in the summer for the lower degree of this in the winter, that it appears to equal the Southern Coast. The mean temperature of the latter during the winter months,* is from one to two degrees above

---

* It may be proper here to state that in this work I adopt the more common division of the seasons; including under *Winter,* the months of December, January, and February; under *Spring,* those of March, April, and May; under *Summer,* June, July, and August; and under *Autumn,* September, October, and November.

that of London. The superiority is greatest in those months in the following order,—January, February, December. This diminishes in March; and in April, the temperature of the coast falls nearly two degrees below that of London and its vicinity; in May, it is a degree and a half less, and in the months of June, July, August, and September, about one degree. In October, the mean temperatures are nearly equal, but in November that of the coast begins to rise above the other.

It is important to remark that the difference of temperature in favour of the coast, occurs principally between the *lower* extremes; so that the temperature of the day is nearly the same at both places, whilst that of the night is considerably warmer on the coast. For instance, the difference between the minima of Gosport and London, during the winter, is to the difference of their maxima as 7 to 3. The minimum temperature observed on the South Coast generally, is from three to four degrees above the minimum temperature observed at London. Nor is the temperature of the South Coast subject to the same extent of range as that of London and the interior. Thus, the difference of the mean temperature of the warmest and coldest months in London is 26°, while at Gosport it is only 21°; and the mean of the monthly ranges at London is 34°, and at Gosport only 31°. In steadiness of climate, as deduced from the variation of temperature between successive days, the South Coast does not appear to possess any very remarkable superiority over London itself. Of the places on this tract of coast which have been particularly examined, Southampton is the most variable in its temperature, equalling in this respect the environs of London.*

A greater quantity of rain falls on the South

---

* In comparing the different places on this line of coast, from observations made during the winters of 1827-8, I find that in *November*, Gosport was two degrees warmer than Hastings and Southampton, and that Southampton was nearly one degree more variable than the other two places. In *December*, Brighton was half a degree warmer than either Hastings or Southampton, and the temperature was much more steady, being less variable than Hastings by a degree and a half, and than Southampton by two degrees and a half. In *January*, Brighton still continued as warm as Southampton, but fell two degrees below Hastings, and two and a half below Gosport; but in steadiness and constancy of temperature it still preserved its superiority over Hastings and Southampton. In *February*, Southampton was the coldest place and also the most variable—Hastings was about half a degree warmer than Brighton—but Gosport the warmest of all. Hastings was less variable in February than the other places. In *March*, Gosport still continued the warmest place, and Hastings was above two degrees warmer than Southampton, which also remained the most variable on the coast. These places would have been compared with each other more minutely had not data been wanting. Gosport is the only place on this coast for which we have complete tables of climate for a series of years.

Coast than at London, the ratio being, as nearly as could be ascertained, as 30 to 25 :—Its distribution we have not been able to obtain with accuracy. Of the different places on this coast frequented by invalids, Hastings, Brighton, and the Isle of Wight may be considered as having, respectively, peculiar climates. All the other places, from Worthing to Southampton, (including Littlehampton, Bognor, Chichester, Portsmouth, and Gosport,) may be classed under another division. The whole tract of country in which these places are situated, is nearly on a level with the sea, which is separated, for the most part, from the chain of hills which traverse the whole of Sussex and Hampshire, by a level and humid plain, from two to ten miles in width. The general character of the climate of this district is humid and heavy ; the hills are generally too distant or too low to afford any protection from winds, and many parts of the plain are subject to aguish complaints. The only places of this division for which we have any thing like accurate registers, for a series of years are Gosport and Chichester, particularly the former ; and the latter place is certainly the best winter residence for that class of invalids likely to be benefited by a climate of this kind.

HASTINGS.

From its low situation and the height of the neighbouring cliffs, this place is protected in a considerable degree from the north and north-easterly winds. " Such is the peculiar situation of Hastings," says Dr. Harwood, " that a considerable portion of it is most securely sheltered by its natural bulwarks from the searching and penetrating agency of these winds."* To the south-west wind it is fully exposed, and although the gales from that quarter are less violent on this coast than on that of Devonshire and Cornwall, still during the winter season they often prevail many days or even weeks together, sometimes very powerfully. " It would be injustice to Hastings," adds Dr. Harwood, " to omit also to notice its very superior suitableness for the employment of exercise in the open air, on the part of invalids, during those months which are usually the most cold and severe. This arises from the peculiar situation of the Parade, which is screened from the before-mentioned (northerly) winds, and the existence of a carriage road, in a more especial manner adapted for this purpose than any other with which I am acquainted on the South coast."

* On the Curative Influence of the Southern Coast of England, especially that of Hastings, &c. By William Harwood, M. D. 1828.

To the westward of Hastings, there is a ride
along the shore, which is well protected from the
north wind, but there is no ride well sheltered
from the east wind. It must be admitted, indeed,
that one of the principal disadvantages of Hastings,
is its confined situation, by which its climate is
limited to a small local extent, owing to the close
manner in which it is hemmed in on the sea by
the steep and high cliffs which rise immediately
behind it.   This circumstance, moreover, gives
the climate of this place a peculiar character
relatively to its effect upon certain constitutions.
With respect to the merits of the climate of
Hastings, it may be observed, that its superiority
in winter appears to be confined chiefly to the
months of January and February, but that during
these and the spring months, it has the advantage
of all the other places frequented on the South
Coast in warmth and shelter from cold winds,
(with the exception, perhaps, of Undercliff, in
the Isle of Wight,) and, consequently, during
this period affords the best residence for those
invalids to whom the climate of this coast is
adapted.   During the autumn months, and even
December, the climate of Brighton appears to be
somewhat warmer and more steady than that of
Hastings.

In its effects on disease, the climate of Hastings
corresponds with that of the South Coast generally ; it is, however, acccording to my experience,

unfavourable in nervous complaints, to persons subject to headache, and to languid or relaxed habits. For persons also who have suffered from ague, I should consider Hastings as a very doubtful residence. There is a degree of closeness and confinement in the atmosphere of the lower and more sheltered parts which is unfavourable to the former class of invalids ; and agues are not unfrequent about Hastings.

BRIGHTON.

The climate of Brighton is, in respect of closeness, the reverse of Hastings ; being dry, elastic and bracing ; and to persons of nervous or relaxed habits, who can bear the sharpness of the cold winds, to which Brighton is fully exposed, it proves a much more congenial climate than the former place. The most favourable season of the year at Brighton is the autumn and beginning of winter ; during this period, as we have already remarked, it appears to be somewhat warmer and more steady than Hastings.

In the case of invalids who are of a relaxed habit, and who suffer from diseases connected with this state of constitution, and are injured by a close or humid state of the atmosphere, and for whom a dry, mild, elastic air is necessary, Brighton, during the autumn, claims the preference over every other place on the coast with which

I am acquainted. The early part of the spring is the worst season at Brighton, its exposure to the north-easterly winds rendering it an unfavourable climate at this season, to all persons disposed to pulmonary or other diseases accompanied with much general or local irritation. As examples of such, I may mention affections of the trachea and bronchia of the dry irritable kind, and dyspepsia arising from an irritated state of the stomach.

For the greater number of valetudinarians who frequent the Southern coast, it is probable that the autumn and beginning of winter may be passed with the greatest advantage at Brighton ;—January and February at Hastings ; and that some sheltered situation in the interior, is preferable to any part of the coast in the spring.

ISLE OF WIGHT.

The only part of this island well adapted as a winter residence for invalids, is that denominated *Undercliff*, which comprehends a tract of country about six miles in length, and from a quarter to half a mile in breadth, situated on the South-East coast, between the villages of Bonchurch and Niton.* This singular district consists of a series of irregular terraces, formed by fragments of rocks

---

* For the following particulars relative to the Isle of Wight I am principally indebted to the kindness of Dr. Lempriere.

of chalk and sandstone, and the alluvia of a rich loam, which have been detached from the cliffs and hills above, and deposited upon a substratum of blue marl. The whole of the Undercliff, which presents in many places scenery of the greatest beauty, is dry and free from moist or impure exhalations, and is completely sheltered from the north, north-east, north-west, and west winds, by a range of lofty downs, or hills, of chalk and sandstone, which rise boldly from the upper termination of these terraces, in elevations varying from four to six and seven hundred feet; leaving Undercliff open only in a direct line to the south-east, and obliquely to the east and south-west winds, which rarely blow here with great force. " On this part of the coast," says Dr. Lempriere, " we have a climate as favorable to the invalid as any part of England can afford. This is proved not only by thermometrical observation, but also by the state of vegetation during the colder months of the year, when the myrtle, geranium, and many other exotic plants flourish luxuriantly in the open air; and that even in seasons when the severity of the frost has destroyed the green-house plants in the north side of the island, although placed in sheltered apartments. Snow is rarely seen, and frosts are only partially felt here."

The mildness of the climate, the dry nature of the soil of Undercliff, and the extent to which it is sheltered from cold winds by affording ample

space for exercise, are great advantages to invalids
threatened with pulmonary disease, or others to
whom exercise in the open air, in a mild climate,
is desirable. In this respect, it is probably superior to any place in this line of coast. The
principal objections to it, as a residence for invalids, are the scantiness of accommodations, and
its distance from medical advice. On this account,
it is perhaps, at present, rather calculated for the
retreat of the valetudinarian, who does not stand
in need of much medical attendance, than for the
real invalid. It is to be regretted that we have no
accurate meteorological observations for Undercliff,
by means of which we might have been able to
compare its climate with that of the more sheltered situations on the south and south-west coasts.

SOUTH-WESTERN COAST.

The south coast of Devon, the warmest part of
this district, has a winter temperature nearly two
degrees higher than that of the coast of Sussex
and Hampshire, and from three to four warmer than
that of London.* During the months of No-

---

* Notwithstanding the public attention has been so long
directed towards the climate of Devonshire, it is extraordinary
how few are the materials which can be collected with a
reference to this subject. It is to be hoped that this may not
long continue to afford a ground of complaint. Why does not
the Western Institution publish its meteorological Journals in
one of the periodical scientific publications, ever ready to receive

vember, December, and January, the difference is most remarkable; amounting, on the average, in the sheltered places, to five degrees above London. In February, the difference falls to three degrees, and in March and April, the excess of the mean temperature over that of London, does not amount to one degree. It ought also to be remarked that this difference takes place principally in the *night;* as the difference between the lower extremes of London and the South-west coast, is to the difference of the higher extremes as 4 to 3,—a less disproportion, however, than occurs between the South coast and London. Hence, when compared with the latter, the days are proportionally warmer on the South-western than on the Southern coast; whilst the nights at both places are nearly equal. The range of daily temperature is about the same on the South-West and South Coasts, although, as has been remarked, less than at London. As regards the continuance of the same temperature the south-western has a remarkable superiority over the southern coast; amounting nearly to

such? And why do not the many intelligent professional men, scattered not thinly over Devonshire, register their observations and lay them before the public? We should think this an object well worth the attention of the scientific Institutions of Exeter, Bath, Bristol, &c. Were they to establish a series of simultaneous observations at different parts of the country for a few years only, the character of the climate of the south-western part of England might be accurately ascertained.

three-fourths of a degree; which is a very considerable difference, when we reflect that the whole amount of variation of successive days scarcely exceeds three degrees.

Different places on the South-West Coast possess these general qualities in a more eminent degree, accordingly as they are more or less sheltered from the north-east wind. Of these *Torquay, Dawlish, Exmouth, Kingsbridge,* and *Salcomb* in the South Hams, (the Montpelier of Huxham,) deserve to be particularly noticed. But many other sheltered spots may be found along this coast, as about *Lyme Regis, Plymouth,* and other places.

TORQUAY.

The general character of the climate of this coast, is soft and humid. Torquay is certainly drier than the other places, and almost entirely free from fogs. This drier state of the atmosphere probably arises, in part, from the lime stone rocks, which are confined to the neighbourhood of this place, and partly from its position between the two streams, the Dart and the Teign, by which the rain is in some degree attracted. Torquay is also very remarkably protected from north-east winds, the great evil of our spring climate. It is likewise well sheltered from the north-west. This protection from winds, extends also over a very considerable tract of beautiful country, abounding in every variety of landscape ; so that there is scarcely a wind that blows, from which the invalid will not be able to find a shelter for exercise either on foot or horseback. In this respect, Torquay is much superior to any other place we have noticed. It possesses all the advantages of the South-Western climate in the highest degree, and, with the exception of its exposure to the south-west gales, (one of the evils of this coast,) partakes less of the disadvantages of it than any other place having accommodations for invalids.* Of the places on this coast frequented by invalids, Dawlish perhaps deserves the preference after Torquay ;— it is less dry and more exposed to easterly winds than the latter place. Exmouth is tolerably well sheltered, but damp and subject to fogs. Sidmouth, as will be perceived by a reference to the tables, possesses very little of the characteristic qualities of this climate. It is open to the valley of the Sid, and exposed to currents of cold wind from the mountains whence this stream takes its rise. It is therefore inferior to all the other places as a winter or spring residence. It may however be an agreeable summer or autumn watering place.

The interior of Devonshire suffers considerably less from violent winds and storms than the coast;

---

* The little village of *Upton*, distant from Torquay only about a mile, would afford one of the best and most favorable situations on this coast for establishing a Madeira village ; being protected from south-west as well as northerly winds.

and, probably, in spring, some of its green sheltered vallies may afford protection from the east winds; but in winter its temperature is considerably lower than that of the coast. It is not unusual to find, a few miles from the sea, hard frost and ice, of which nothing is known at Torquay, and the comparison of the temperature of this place with that of Totness, (distant only about 20 miles) is very unfavorable to the latter.

The climate of the coast of Devonshire is found very beneficial in various forms of disease. I have known it serviceable in chronic affections of the throat, trachea and bronchia, proceeding from irritation, or a low degree of inflammation of these parts, and attended with a dry cough, or with little expectoration; likewise, in an irritable or morbidly sensitive state of the stomach, and in hypochondriacal affections, the consequence of such a state. In dysmenorrhœa and all nervous sympathetic affections dependant on that disorder; in a highly sensitive state of the nervous system, and in most diseases of general irritation, advantage may be expected from this climate. On the other hand, it certainly exerts an unfavourable influence on nervous headachs, and on all nervous complaints arising from relaxation or want of tone of the nervous system; it is injurious also in pure dyspepsia, when the tone and sensibility of the stomach are below par, as indicated by pale lips, a pale clammy state of the tongue, and languid circulation; and it will be found no less unfavorable in menorrhagia, in leucorrhœa, and all diseases accompanied with much general relaxation of the system, or with much discharge from the affected organs.

What may be the real estimation in which the climate ought to be held in consumptive complaints, and what may be its absolute effect upon these, I have much difficulty in saying; but this much I may venture to advance, that as the invalid will be exposed to less rigorous cold, and for a shorter season,—will have more hours of fine weather, and, consequently, more exercise in the open air,—he gives himself a better chance by passing the winter here, than he could have in any more northern part of our Island. To compare it, also, in this respect, with the climate of the southern continent of Europe, is no easy task. In the South, the invalid has finer days, a drier air, and more constant weather; but the transitions of temperature, though less frequent, are more considerable. In the nights I believe invalids are often exposed to severer cold than here; and this arises partly from the great range of temperature, and partly from the imperfect manner they are protected from the cold of night, by the bad arrangement of the houses, chimnies, &c. To afford an opportunity of judging of the proper value of this last circumstance, I subjoin a comparison of the temperature in-doors and out-of-doors, from observations made by the same invalid

(a correct and careful observer) at Nice and Torquay.* I am possessed of similar observations for
Rome, but they were not made with such precautions as to admit of their being fairly compared
with these.

CORNWALL.

There are several places both on the north and
south coasts of the extended Cornish peninsula,
that would deserve attention in an inquiry like the
present. But here, as elsewhere, the scantiness
and imperfection of our meteorological data, greatly
circumscribe our investigations. Accordingly, the
only places of which I am enabled to speak with
some confidence, are one or two near the south-
western extremity of the peninsula.

PENZANCE.

This place, for various reasons, claims a distinct notice in this work. It is situated on the
coast, on the shore of the beautiful *Mount's-Bay*,
about ten miles from the extreme western point
of England, termed the Land's-end. Penzance,
although situated on the shore of a bay surrounded
by high land, can hardly be said to be sheltered
from any wind; it therefore exhibits, in its meteorological results, the common features of the district
in which it lies. Dr. Forbes was the first to point

* See Table on the opposite page.

ACCOUNT OF THE TEMPERATURE EXPERIENCED BY AN INVALID CONFINED TO THE HOUSE AT NICE AND TORQUAY, COMPARED WITH THE TEMPERATURE OF THE EXTERNAL AIR.

	Exposure of Apartments	NOVEMBER Mean Temp.	Nov. Monthly	Nov. Daily	Nov. Var. Mean	Nov. Var. Extreme	DECEMBER Mean Temp.	Dec. Monthly	Dec. Daily	Dec. Var. Mean	Dec. Var. Extreme	JANUARY Mean Temp.	Jan. Monthly	Jan. Daily	Jan. Var. Mean	Jan. Var. Extreme	FEBRUARY Mean Temp.	Feb. Monthly	Feb. Daily	Feb. Var. Mean	Feb. Var. Extreme	MARCH Mean Temp.	Mar. Monthly	Mar. Daily	Mar. Var. Mean	Mar. Var. Extreme	APRIL Mean Temp.	Apr. Monthly	Apr. Daily	Apr. Var. Mean	Apr. Var. Extreme
NICE 1896-7	SOUTH Internal Temp. [Fire only at night.]	59.94	13	3	1.70	3	60.89	10	4	0.93	5	55.28	14	3	1.60	6	58.72	9	4	1.06	5	62.70	7	2	0.79	3	63.40	6	1	0.63	2
	External Temp.	53.70	18	6	1.90	17	48.60	19	6	2.40	14	45.85	31	6	2.60	8	49.00	21	9	3.0	12	51.45	24	9	2.40	8	57.00	23	11	4.00	8
TORQUAY 1897-8	NORTH Internal Temp. [Fire almost constantly.]	63.90	7	1	0.83	4	64.52	6	2	0.83	4	63.56	6	1	0.78	4	62.60	11	3	1.08	7	63.16	9	3	0.85	8	64.64	6	2	0.76	5
	External Temp.	49.90	29	5	3.50	19	48.36	18	5	4.00	14	45.91	25	5	3.40	11	45.48	29	6	3.45	11	48.20	23	8	3.20	18	62.82	26	11	2.50	9

out the character of this climate ; * and in the
course of my survey of other climates, I have
found every reason for considering it as very peculiar, and indeed unlike any other which I have
met with. It would have spared me much trouble
and time, had I had the facility afforded me, in
other climates, for which we are indebted to Dr.
Forbes in regard to this. A few such analyses, as
his "Observations" present, would soon make the
problem of the climate of this country, as regards
all useful purposes, cease to be a desideratum.

The mean annual temperature of Penzance is
52°.16, being only 1°.77 above that of London.
But this temperature is very differently distributed
over the year at the two places. Although Penzance is only a degree and a half warmer than
London for the whole year, it is $5\frac{1}{2}°$ warmer in
winter. It is 2° colder in summer ; scarcely one
degree warmer in the spring; and only about $2\frac{1}{2}°$
warmer in the autumn.

As regards the temperature of the different
months, relatively with London, the greatest difference occurs in the following order,—December,
January, November and February. In April, the
difference is reduced to half a degree ; in May,
Penzance is a degree colder than London, and
in July it is $2\frac{1}{2}°$ colder ; and the temperature does

---

* See Observations on the Climate of Penzance and the
District of the Land's-end : by John Forbes, M. D. 1821.

not again rise above that of London until the
month of October. So that were one to give a
graphical term of expression for the progression
of the mean temperature of the two places through
the year, that of London would more resemble an
ellipsis, and that of Penzance the more equal
figure of a circle. This will be aptly illustrated
by observing that the difference between the mean
temperature of the warmest and coldest months
in London is 26°, while at Penzance it is only 18°;
and that, whilst in London the mean difference
of the temperature of successive months is 4°.36,
it is only 3° at Penzance. On examining the progression of temperature for the twenty-four hours
at these two places, we find that, in winter, it is
during the night that the greater part of this difference of temperature occurs; Penzance being
nearly, on an average, six degrees and a half
warmer than London during the night; and only
little more than three degrees warmer during the
day. This distinction ought to afford matter for
the physician's consideration. But this equal distribution of heat throughout the year at Penzance,
which we have compared so advantageously with
that of London, is still more striking when compared with that of the South of Europe. Madeira
is the only climate which we have examined that
is superior to Penzance in this quality.

The same remarkable equality in the distribution
of temperature through the year at Penzance,

holds equally true for the day;* and, indeed, I may observe generally, that the progression of temperature for the year and the day, are faithful types of each other. I find, on comparing the months for a series of years, that the daily range at Penzance is almost half that of the South of Europe ; but in this quality, also, it falls short of Madeira. And here is a proper opportunity of remarking, that although in mean temperature for all the twenty-four hours, Penzance is considerably lower than that of the South of Europe, yet that during the night, through the winter, its extreme minimum temperature falls seldom so low as that of the former climate. It is during the day only that the South of Europe, as far as regards temperature simply, possesses a superiority. Thus in winter, at seven o'clock in the morning, there is little difference between Rome and Penzance, but at two o'clock in the afternoon there is nearly the difference of 7°. Indeed the whole advantage of Penzance, as compared with the South of Europe, appears to occur in the winter during the night.†

* Thus in the winter of 1827-8, the mean daily range at Penzance was $7^b.50$; at London, at Gosport, Torquay, and Nice, it was 12°, 10°, 11°, and 11° respectively.

† In the winter of 1827-8, the lower extreme of Penzance is 2°.40 above that of Torquay ; whilst its higher extreme is only 1°.50 ; at Gosport, the former is 2°.10 and the latter 1°.50 ; at Nice, the lower extreme is nearly the same as at Penzance, but the higher is on an average 3°.30 above that of Penzance.

In the duration of the same temperature, as shown by the mean variation of successive days, the climate of Penzance excels all the northern climates, and nearly equals Rome and Nice in this respect; but as compared with Madeira, its temperature from day to day varies twice as much.*

As will have been observed, Penzance loses in the spring its superiority of climate. In April and May, it appears decidedly inferior to the South-Western Coast, and very much so to the South-West of France. For instance, at *Pau*, the mean

---

* With the view of giving a general idea of the difference of temperature, during part of the year, between Penzance and the South of Europe, on the one hand, and the South of Scotland on the other, the following statement is subjoined:

	Temperature of Rome higher than that of Penzance by	Temperature of Penzance higher than that of Kinfauns (near Perth) by
December	3°	8°
January	5°	3°
February	5°	4°.6
March	6°	7°.8
Winter	3°	5°
Spring	8°	5°

The high temperature of *Kinfauns* in January, which is even above that of London, is remarkable, when contrasted with the other winter and spring months; yet the same thing occurs at *Leith*, as may be seen by a reference to the tables on climate. I cannot help doubting whether this would be the case in a series of years.

temperature during the winter is nearly 3° below that of Penzance, while during the spring it is 5° above it.

In the other elements of climate, this district has less peculiar advantages. There falls at Penzance nearly twice as much rain as at London, the annual average at the former place being 44 and at the latter only 25 inches. We have reason to believe also that the number of days in which rain falls is greater at Penzance than at London, although this is not the result of Mr. Giddy's observations as given in his tables.* Dr. Forbes, however, who had ample means of forming a correct judgment, inclines to our opinion, and his testimony is extremely strong in respect of the humidity of the air. " Cornwall," he says, " has been ever obnoxious to the charge of great hu-

---

* In Mr. Giddy's tables the number of rainy days is only 170, being less by eight than London. We suspect that Mr. Giddy only recorded as rainy days such as paid tribute to his rain-gauge. Now we know by experience that many days deserve the appellation of rainy (in a medical point of view at least) in which none is deposited in the gauge. And this we apprehend is peculiarly the case with the Land's-end district. At Helston too, which is only twelve miles distant from Penzance, Mr. Moyle gives the average number of rainy days as 195 ; but perhaps there may be something in the topographical relations of the former place that will account for more days of actual rain. In the year 1821, according to Dr. Forbes' own register, the fall of rain was 46.20 inches, and the number of rainy days 179 at Penzance.

midity; and in as far as the charge rests on hygrometrical humidity, and also on the number of days on which rain falls, perhaps it is well founded. I am unacquainted with any hygrometrical observations that have been made in this part of the country; I cannot therefore give any precise statement either of the comparative or actual humidity of its atmosphere. There can be no doubt, however, that this is much greater than in the interior counties. Its situation alone may be deemed sufficient to prove this; but the fact is further demonstrated by many well known peculiarities. There is much greater difficulty, for instance, of guarding against the oxydation of iron at Penzance than at London, a fact well known and admitted by every one here resident. The great prevalence of westerly winds in this district will be more particularly noticed hereafter. Now this wind, if it does not *always* bring rain, certainly has always qualities of great humidity, sufficiently cognizable to our senses. Our warm west winds often bring with them a sort of drizzly rain, sufficient to wet thoroughly grass and other vegetables, or the clothes of a person exposed to it; while neither the rain-gauge, nor the roads nor streets, show any indication of its presence, unless long continued."* Another of the disadvantages of the climate of the south-western extremity of our Island,

* Op. Cit., pp. 25, 26.

is its liability to violent and frequent storms of
wind, and of this disadvantage Penzance appears
to partake largely. Carew, as quoted by Dr.
Forbes, states that " the country is much subject
to storms, which fetching a large course in the
open sea, do from thence violently assault the
dwellers at land, and leave them uncovered
houses, pared hedges, and dwarf trees, as wit-
nesses of their force and fury." " Dr. Borlase,"
says Dr. Forbes, " gives the same account of the
frequency and violence of the storms and squalls
in Cornwall, and my own experience leads me to
the same conclusion. Indeed, I think the climate
of the west of Cornwall is fully as remarkable
for its great variability in respect of wind and
rain, as it is for the singular unchangeableness
of its temperature."* During the spring the
northerly and easterly winds are the most prevalent, which circumstance sufficiently accounts
for the lower temperature of that season ; though,
as Dr. Forbes remarks, the effects of these winds
as indicated by the thermometer are much_less
than our sensations would lead us to expect.
" It may be stated," he says " as a general
fact, that the south and west winds are uniformly
warm and soft, and the north and east winds
uniformly cold and sharp. These unvarying effects on sensation are as certainly, although in

* Op. cit., p. 37, 38.

a lesser degree, indicated by the thermometer.
In the winter and spring months, the north and
east winds may be considered as having a temperature 6° or 8° lower than the south and west
winds; and this is so constant a result, that the
change of temperature is as regular as the change
of the wind."*

The frequency and severity of the winds at
Penzance constitute one of the greatest disadvantages of its climate; and it is principally in
consequence of its exposure to those from the
north-east during the spring months, that it is
absolutely colder than the coast of Devonshire,
or even the neighbourhood of Bristol, during this
season. This circumstance of exposure to, or
shelter from cold winds, constitutes the principal
cause of the difference of different places, in the
same line of climate, in point of warmth as
experienced by man; for the influence of temperature on the living body is indicated more
accurately by our sensations than by the thermometer. Unless, therefore, the indications of
the thermometer are corrected by observing the
winds, we shall form very erroneous ideas of the
climate of many places.

The effects of the southerly winds at Penzance
are widely different. " During the prevalence of
the south or south-west gales," says Dr. Forbes,

* Op. cit., p. 37, 38.

" there is very little difference of temperature
between the day and night, as proved by the
register thermometer. Sometimes there is no
difference whatever; and very commonly the
minimum of the night is not more than 3° or 4°
below the maximum of the day. This shows how
very completely the influence of the sun is ex-
cluded by the dense vapour with which the air
is loaded; and during these *our moist siroccos,*
we may say, without any metaphor, that we are
breathing the breezes of a climate milder than our
own. When these south and south-west winds,
so prevalent in winter, are very gentle, the sky
is often clear for many days together. On these
occasions, the warmth and softness of the air are
truly delightful; and when taken in conjunction
with the beautiful scenery around Penzance,—the
calm blue bay,—the gay green meadows,—the
myrtles, and other exotic plants common in our
shrubberies,—one is almost tempted to forget that
it is a British and winter landscape that he is
contemplating."

The only other place in this district that deserves notice is *Falmouth,* including the neighbouring village of *Flushing.* The winter temperature of Falmouth (which lies about thirty
miles to the east of Penzance) is a trifle lower
than that of the latter place, but the general
qualities of its climate are nearly the same. In
one respect, indeed, the village of Flushing, which

is situated on the east side of the river Fal,
(Falmouth being on the west,) has the advantage
of Penzance, being much better sheltered from
the east winds by the hills which rise immediately
above it. If it possessed good accommodations,
erected in the best point, this village would form
a residence for invalids, during the spring months,
much superior to Penzance.

With respect to the effects of the climate of the
Land's-end on disease, the disadvantages which
attach to it generally, in point of humidity and
exposure to winds, are such, as in a great measure
to neutralize the superiority which it possesses over
the other climates of England in mildness and
equability of temperature. In its general characters, this climate resembles so closely that of
the south coast of Devonshire, that the remarks
formerly made on the influence of the latter on
disease, apply nearly to it. Regarding its influence
on consumption, we have the testimony of Dr.
Forbes, founded on ample experience, that little
is to be expected from it; but we ought to admit,
at the same time, that, in this respect, it but shares
the opprobium with every other climate, in the
advanced stages of that disease. " During are si-
dence of five years," says Dr. Forbes, " at Penzance, in Cornwall, a place much frequented by
consumptive patients on account of the extreme
mildness and equability of its temperature, I had
extensive opportunities of observing the effect of

change of climate in phthisis; and I am sorry to say that, in the greater number of cases, the change was not beneficial. This result, however, must not, in fairness, be considered as derogating, in any considerable degree, either from the propriety of the practice, or the fitness of the situation; since it must be confessed that few of the invalids came to Penzance in that period of the disease when a cure could be expected, if indeed it were even possible. In no case of well marked tubercular phthisis did I witness a cure, or even a temporary alleviation, that could fairly be attributed to change of climate. In a good many cases, however, of chronic bronchitis, simulating phthisis, the health was greatly improved, and in some it was completely restored, from a state of great debility and seeming danger. In a few cases, also, of young persons who accompanied their diseased relatives, and in whom the hereditary predisposition was strongly marked, if there was not already evidence of nascent tubercles,—a great and striking improvement in the general health and strength followed within a short period after their arrival, and seemed fairly attributable to the combined influence of change of air, scene and habits." *

The consumptive cases in which the soft humid atmosphere of this place is likely to prove bene-

* Dr. Forbes' Translation of Laennec's Treatise on Diseases of the Chest. Note by translator, 3d Edit. p. 73.

ficial, are those in which the disease is accompanied with an irritated state of the mucous membrane of the lungs, producing a dry cough, or one with little expectoration.

In idiopathic tracheal and bronchial diseases of the same character, whether complicated with asthma, or otherwise, and also in certain pure cases of the latter disease, it is likely to be very beneficial. When, on the contrary, there exists a relaxed state of the general system, or a disposition to copious secretion from the bronchial membrane, whether idiopathic or symptomatic of a tuberculous state of the lungs, or where hæmoptysis has occurred, I believe the climate of the Land's-end will generally prove injurious.

As a summer residence for invalids, and also as a residence for the whole year, I consider the district of the Land's-end superior to the coast of Devonshire. In the winter, however, and still more especially in the spring, the latter will, I believe, in most cases, deserve a preference. If Penzance is somewhat warmer and more equable in its temperature, it is more humid and more exposed to storms during the winter, whilst it is rather colder, and less protected from the northeast winds during the spring. Many aged invalids, to whom in general humidity is less objectionable, might more particularly derive advantage by residing the whole year at Penzance. The great mildness of the winter would enable them to be much in the open air, and they would have less to dread from the coldness of the nights than in any other part of England.

The country around Penzance is healthy, and affords a great variety of excellent rides and drives. Accommodations for invalids are numerous; and being a sea-port, the place affords convenience for water exercise during the summer. Invalids who have passed the winter at Penzance, and whose complaints are likely to be aggravated by the spring winds, might remove to Flushing at that season; or some might even go to Clifton with advantage.*

WEST OF ENGLAND.

I regret not having found it possible to procure more information on that tract of country which extends along the Bristol Channel from Wells to Gloucester. We are in possession of observations for a series of years for Clifton and Cheltenham only, and these are very imperfect. Those for the

---

* For much interesting information respecting the natural history and antiquities of this district, I refer the reader to Dr. Forbes' tract, so often quoted above, and to an amusing little work, entitled, " *A Guide to Penzance and the Land's End*," written, it is said, by an eminent physician now resident in London.

winter of 1827-8, for Bath, Bristol and Cheltenham, seem more to be depended on.*

The mean temperature of the western groupe of climates, during the winter, is rather lower than that of the Southern Coast, but in March and April rises rather above it. The mean annual temperature of Cheltenham appears to be about one degree warmer than London ; its winter, spring and summer, from one to two degrees warmer ; but its autumn somewhat colder. Bath and Bristol, during the months of November and December, are nearly 3° warmer than London. In January and February they do not average one degree warmer ; in March, Bath and Cheltenham are rather colder than London, but Bristol continues from one to two degrees warmer during March as well as April. During the months of November and December of 1827, the mean temperature of Bristol fell only one degree below Torquay ; in January 2°, in February 1°, and in March and April it rose somewhat higher.

---

* Finding it so difficult to obtain observations on the climates of different places for a series of years, I procured as many as I could for 1827-8, in order that I might be able to compare them with each other. Observations for a single year cannot, of course, be relied on as affording data on which to found a permanent character of a climate.. Fortunately, however, this year was generally a very mild and equable one over the whole country, and was therefore favourable for comparing the different places with each other, if not for fixing the climate of these respectively.

With Bath and Cheltenham the difference was more considerable; and even in March and April they continued from 2° to 3° below Torquay. On comparing Penzance with this tract, we find only 1° of difference in the mean annual temperature. In winter, however, Penzance is 4° warmer; but in the spring and summer it is somewhat colder.* With regard to the distribution of heat throughout the year, we find it more unequal in this district than in the others examined; the difference of the warmest and coldest months being 28°, while it is only 26° at London, 21° at Gosport, 20° at Torquay, and 18° at Penzance. We find, also, that although the range of temperature for the day and the month is less than at London, it is considerably more than on the Southern, South-western coasts, and Land's-end; the minimum term of temperature falling from 3° to 5°, and even 6° lower than at some of these places. In steadiness of temperature from day to day, it offers very little advantage over London; and in this respect nearly corresponds with the South Coast, but is inferior to the Coast of Devon, and considerably

---

* In 1827-8, Penzance was in November 2° warmer than Bristol, and 4° warmer than Bath and Cheltenham; in December, 1½° above Bristol, and 3½° above Bath and Cheltenham; in January, 4° warmer than Bristol, and 5° than the other places; in February, only 1½° warmer than Bristol; in March, ½°, and in April, 1½° colder.

so to Penzance. " Great Britain," says Dr. Chisholm, " presents almost the extreme of irregularity in her climate ; and probably the western counties are the most distinguished for that versatility, that capriciousness of temperature so peculiar to the whole of England."*

Part of this tract of country is traversed by the elevated ridge of Mendip, which rises on the edge of the Bristol channel, and crosses the county from West to East The district on the southern side of this chain of hills, Mr. Mansford thinks, affords one of the most favourable residences for those disposed to consumptive diseases which our Island affords. " A salutary retreat," he says, " may here be found at all seasons of the year, and especially during the winter and spring months, from the mildness of the air, and the shelter afforded by the Mendip hills ; which, like a stupendous wall towards the North and North-east, afford an effectual screen to the winds blowing from those points, which, especially in the spring, are generally the most prevalent."†

In this tract of country, the vicinity of Bristol and Clifton appears to afford the most eligible

* See an excellent paper on the statistical pathology of Bristol and Clifton, by the late Dr. Chisholm.—*Ed. Med. and Surg. Journal*, Vol. xiii. 1817.

† An Inquiry into the influence of situation on Pulmonary Consumption, &c., by John G. Mansford, p. 54.

winter and spring residence for invalids. At the bottom of the hill in the neighbourhood of the Bristol Hotwells, the most sheltered situations are to be found. Of this place, the late Dr. Nott remarks,—" To no spot in our kingdom can the valetudinarian fly, or can the physician consign his patient, for a re-establishment of health impaired by disease, where the purpose is more attainable, than in the neighbourhood of St. Vincent's Rock. The upland habitations on Clifton Hill during the summer are delightful; and the sheltered situation of those round the Hotwells below, afford a warm residence in winter, equal at least to the boasted Coast of Devonshire; indeed it has one advantage over it, being free from its damp airs and mizzling rains."* " Had Dr. Nott," observes Dr. Chisholm, " adverted to the influence of subincumbent lime stone, as constituting the salubrity of the atmosphere, his picture would have been more complete. The absence of every thing like marsh must certainly contribute greatly to the purity and wholesomeness of the Clifton air." " In the list of diseases admitted during four years into the dispensary, only one case of intermittent fever appeared, and that one was from the fenny district near Conglesbury, about twelve miles to the westward of

* Of the Hotwell Waters near Bristol, by John Nott, M. D. 1793.

Clifton." "The whole parish of Clifton," Dr. Chisholm further adds, "is a beautiful and romantic assemblage of woods, rock, water, pasture and down. It seems indeed singularly well adapted to the maintenance of health; the soil resting on immense beds of lime-stone rock, exposed to the southerly and westerly winds, for nearly three fourths of the year; with an atmosphere elastic, vivifying—not humid."*

From all these testimonies in favour of the climate of the more sheltered parts about Bristol and Clifton, there appears sufficient evidence of this spot being the mildest winter, and more especially spring residence, in the West of England. This results also from its sheltered situation, and the evidence afforded by our meteorological registers, which, we have seen, make Bristol warmer than the South Coast, and equalling that of Devonshire during the spring months. This country affords also a good summer climate; so that for invalids to whom the air of this district is suitable, it presents altogether one of the best residences throughout the whole year in our Island. The valetudinarian should seek the lower and more protected situations about the Hotwells during the winter and spring, and the more ele-

* The average quantity of rain for six years is 31 inches, about the same as falls on the South Coast; London is 25 inches.

vated places on Clifton Hill in the summer; or a change to the more interior parts of the country, as to Cheltenham, or still better, to Malvern, may be in many cases adviseable. In other cases, the summer months may be passed in South Wales; and in such chronic complaints as a course of goat's whey promises benefit, this will be the best place. But the preference to be given to either of these situations must of course depend on the nature of the individual case. It may however be stated, that when a change of air can be made during the summer months, it will generally prove beneficial to the invalid; although the amount of benefit will depend, in a great measure, upon the fitness of the summer residence selected.

In bringing to a conclusion this brief account of the warmer situations in our own Island, it may naturally be expected that I should apply the preceding observations on the physical characters of their climates to the object of our researches; and say what are the advantages which they hold out generally to invalids; and what are the diseases in which they are respectively beneficial.

The whole of these places, as we have seen, are considerably warmer during the winter and spring than England generally, and much warmer than the colder parts of it. Indeed, as I have shown, and as a reference to the tables on climate will further prove, there exists as much difference between the temperature, and its distribution, in the south of Scotland and south of England, as between the latter and the south of Europe. Now as the influence of temperature on the living body is, in a great degree, relative, an inhabitant of one of the coldest parts of our island would, it is reasonable to believe, feel the influence of the climate of the south-west of England (as far, at least, as regards temperature) as much as an inhabitant of the latter would that of the south of Europe.* An invalid, therefore, from the northern parts of England, or from Scotland, will find in the places we have pointed out, a milder climate during the winter and spring, that

* The influence of relative temperature on organic life might be aptly illustrated by a reference to its very remarkable effects on plants ; and the influence of warmth, whether natural or artificial, in exciting or accelerating the vegetation of these, affords matter for the reflection of the physician in estimating the effects of climate on man. It is, I believe, a general practice with gardeners in respect to plants, which they wish to force rapidly in the hot-house, to keep them previously in as cold a temperature as they will bear. And it has been often proved, that a vine accustomed to the temperature of the open air, will vegetate in winter if transferred to the hot-house, while a plant from the same stock, accustomed to the stove, will remain without any sign of budding.

is to say, he will be exposed to a less degree of cold, and for a shorter period; and he will, in consequence, be enabled to take much more exercise in the open air, than he could have done at home.

But it must be kept in mind, that, as has been before observed, there are other circumstances connected with the adaptation of climate to disease, which require attention, as well as temperature. The particular nature of the disease and of the patient's constitution, and the character of the climate most suitable for these, will naturally be the first objects of the physician's consideration; but the nature of the climate in which the invalid has lived, ought also to be taken into account. This last circumstance, namely, the comparative influence of any particular climate on different individuals, depending on the nature of that which they previously inhabited, has not, I believe, been sufficiently attended to. It deserves, however, the especial consideration of physicians when selecting a climate for their patients.

With respect to the merits of the milder parts of England in their influence on disease, I have already made a few remarks while treating of particular places. As regards consumptive invalids, for whom climate has been looked to as

the great resource, I beg to refer the reader to
the article on Consumption, in a subsequent part
of this volume; and to what has been already
said on this subject, while noticing the climates
of Devonshire and the Land's-end. I may
remark here, that it is (with a few exceptions
only) as a means of preventing the occurrence
of tuberculer disease in the lungs, when threatened, or of checking its progress in its early
stages, that much benefit can be expected from
any climate. With this view, the preference to
be given to any of the milder situations in England, in such cases, must depend greatly on the
nature of the person's constitution, and partly also
on the other morbid states with which the consumptive tendency may be complicated. Keeping
these circumstances (the whole of which have
been noticed in the articles referred to) in mind,
the situation which admits of the invalid's being
most in the open air without risk from cold,
should in general be preferred. The selection
will, I believe, lie among the following places, as
winter and spring residences,—Torquay, Undercliff, Hastings and Clifton; and perhaps, in the
generality of cases, they will deserve the preference
in the order stated. But I wish to be understood
as speaking with much diffidence on this subject.

In diseases depending upon, or connected with,

much general or local irritation; in chronic inflammatory affections of the throat, trachea and
bronchia, accompanied with little secretion or
expectoration ; in indigestion, arising from a
heated and irritated state of the stomach, and
in the nervous and hypochondriacal affections
originating in such a state; in dysmenorrhœa,
and in dry irritable cutaneous diseases, the coast
of Devonshire affords the most favourable winter
climate. In cases of the kind referred to, in
which it is desirable that the invalid should
remain stationary during the whole year, the
Land's-end would perhaps be preferable to the
coast of Devon.

In chronic diseases of the trachea and bronchia,
on the other hand, which are attended with
copious expectoration and dyspnœa; in dyspeptic
disorders of a more purely nervous character,
and where there is a relaxed state of the system,
or a tendency to copious mucous or sanguineous
discharges, the climates of the South-West of
England and the Land's-end are unfavourable.
It is indeed difficult to find any place in our
island, the climate of which is very suitable for
such cases, during the whole of the cold season.
Brighton is, I believe, the most favourable residence during the autumn and early part of the
winter. The climate of this place is generally

mild and equable, and the air comparatively dry
and elastic at this season.* But during the later
part of the winter, and still more in the spring,
Brighton is cold, being exposed to all the severity
of the north-east winds. Hastings is then considerably warmer and more sheltered. The neighbourhood of Bristol and Clifton affords a good
spring residence in the affections which we have
noticed ; but the distance from the South Coast
will render such a change in general unadviseable,
as well as inconvenient. Invalids labouring under
the chronic affections mentioned, and who cannot
absent themselves from London during the whole
season, might go to Brighton during the autumn
and early part of winter, remain in town in the
winter, and go to Clifton in the spring ; or,
should this be inconvenient, Chelsea and Brompton
afford sheltered spring situations, which might
be found suitable.

When we are better acquainted with the climates of the warmest and more sheltered parts
of Sussex, of Surrey, and Hampshire, a better
and more convenient arrangement, I have no
doubt, may be made for such patients. On the
present occasion, however, it was with difficulty
I could collect materials for determining with

---

* In disorders of the digestive organs, the water of Brighton
frequently disagrees ; persons suffering from indigestion should
therefore drink distilled water when there.

some accuracy the characters of the principal
places in this country resorted to by invalids;
and this, I hope, may be received as an apology
for the meagre account of them with which I
have been obliged to content myself. It is right,
moreover, to add, that my experience of the
effects of these climates on diseases is still too
limited to enable me to speak of their remedial
qualities in the same decided manner, which
I feel warranted in doing respecting most places
frequented by invalids in the south of Europe.

———

FRANCE.

⸻

THE South of France has been long held in estimation for the mildness of its winter climate, and various parts of it have been and are still annually resorted to by invalids from this country; although, I fear, without much discrimination, either as regards the qualities of the climate, or the nature of the diseases in which this is most likely to prove beneficial.

The climate of the Southern provinces of France admit of being classed under two divisions,— namely, the South-eastern and South-western. These two regions differ essentially from each other in the physical characters of their climates: the latter resembles in its general qualities the South-western parts of England, the former is of a totally different nature. In their influence on disease they differ also in a very remarkable manner; and unless the distinctive characters of each, in this respect, be kept in view by the physician, in selecting a residence in this country for invalids, great errors must be committed.

THE WEST AND SOUTH-WEST
OF FRANCE.

Under this title I include the whole tract of
country from Brittany to Bayonne, comprising
L'Orient, Nantes, La Rochelle, Bourdeaux, Mon-
tauban, Pau, and Toulouse. The islands of Guern-
sey and Jersey also belong to this range of climate;
or they may be considered as intermediate between
that of the South-West of France and England.

The climate of this part of France resembles,
as has been just observed, that of the South-West
of England; while it is, on the other hand, directly opposed, in its qualities, to that of the
South-East of France. Though, on the whole,
less warm than the latter, its temperature is more
equal, and the range of this less extensive, as well
through the whole year, as through the period of
day and night. It is, however, more changeable
from day to day, and the changes themselves are
very considerable. The mean annual temperature
of the South-West of France generally, is about
55°. This makes it 6° higher than England generally, and 4° higher than the south-west of
England; but 3° below the south-east of France,
and 4° below Italy. The days are not so fine as
in the south-eastern parts of the kingdom, but the
nights are not so cold in relation to the days.
The climate may be characterized as soft, relaxing,

and rather wet. Hence it is suitable for complaints to which the south-east of France is injurious, particularly gastritic dyspepsia, (or dyspepsia depending on an inflammatory state of the stomach,) and the dry bronchial irritations. In that class of consumptive patients, therefore, in whom the disease is complicated with either or both of these affections, and in whom, consequently, there is a great susceptibility to the influence of dry, keen winds, this climate will generally agree. Laennec found the southern coast of Brittany very favourable to consumptive patients; and he also observed that the proportion of consumptive diseases in this part of France, was comparatively small.

The climate of this coast is very mild during the winter and temperate during the summer. "From observations made in Brittany for twelve years, at St. Malo, at Nantes, and at Brest, the mean temperature of this peninsula appears to be above 56°.3. In the interior of France, where the land is not much elevated above the sea, we must descend 3° of latitude in order to find an annual temperature like this.

" In the Department of Finisterre, the arbutus, the pomegranate-tree, the *Yucca gloriosa* and *aloifolia;* the *Erica Mediterranea,* the *Hortensia,* the *Fuchsia,* the *Dahlia,* resist in open ground the inclemency of a winter which lasts scarcely fifteen or twenty days, and which succeeds to a summer

F

by no means warm. During this short winter, the thermometer sometimes falls to 17°.6. The sap ascends in the trees from the month of February; but it often freezes even in the middle of May. The *Lavatera Arborea* is found wild in the isle of Glenans, and opposite to this island, on the continent, the *Astragalus Bajonensis*, and the *Laurus nobilis*."*

Generally speaking, the climate of the South-West of France will be useful in chronic inflammatory affections of the mucous membranes accompanied with little secretion, as in chronic bronchitis not attended by much expectoration, or difficulty of breathing, and in similar morbid states of the larynx and trachea. It will be equally proper in dry scaly eruptions of the skin; in dysmenorrhæa; in certain kinds of headach, especially those induced or exasperated by sharp north-east winds; and in high morbid sensibility in general, when accompanied with that habit of body which the ancients called ·*strictum*. On the other hand, the same diseases occurring in relaxed habits in which there is a disposition to copious secretion, will be increased by this climate. Those who do not find inconvenience from the south-west winds of Devonshire, will find the climate agreeable.

* Bonnemaison, *Geogr. Botan. du Depart. de Finisterre*, (*Journal de Botan.*, tom. iii., p. 118,) as cited by Humboldt, on Isothermal Lines.

PAU.

Pau, the capital of the Department of the lower Pyrenees, and the only place in this district of which I consider it necessary to give a particular account, is finely situated upon a ridge of gravelly hills, overlooking an extensive valley to the north. The Pyrenees rise gradually behind it, their higher range being nearly forty miles distant. Pau is about 150 miles distant from Bourdeaux, and 50 from Bayonne. Having made but a short visit to this place myself, I am principally indebted for the following account of it to the kindness of Dr. Playfair, (now of Florence,) who resided there for several years.

Although the character of the climate of Pau corresponds with that of the south-west of France generally, it possesses some peculiarities which it owes to its topographical situation. Notwithstanding its distance from the coast, it is very much under the influence of the Atlantic. All the changes to which this gives rise extend as far as Pau, though modified, in some degree, by distance, and, still more, by the position of the place with respect to the neighbouring mountains. Calmness, for example, is a striking character of the climate, high winds being of rare occurrence and of short duration.

The mean annual temperature of Pau is $4\frac{1}{2}°$

higher than that of London, and about 3° higher
than that of Penzance; it is about 5° lower than
that of Marseilles, Nice and Rome, and 10° lower
than that of Madeira. In *winter*, it is 2° warmer
than London, 3° colder than Penzance, 6° colder
than Nice and Rome, and 18° colder than Madeira. But in the *spring*, Pau is 6° warmer than
London, and 5° warmer than Penzance; only
$2\frac{1}{2}$° colder than Marseilles and Rome, and 7°
colder than Madeira. The range of temperature
between the warmest and coldest months at Pau
is 32°; this at London, and likewise at Rome,
is 26°; at Penzance it is only 18°, and at Madeira, 14°. The daily range of temperature at
Pau is $7\frac{1}{2}$°; at Penzance it is $6\frac{1}{2}$°; at Nice, $8\frac{1}{2}$°;
at Rome, 11°.

The annual quantity of rain has not been
measured at Pau. The number of days in which
rain falls is 109, nearly the same as at Rome,
and about 70 less than at London. The west
wind, blowing directly from the Atlantic, is accompanied with rain; the wind from the north-
west, and from this point to the north-east, brings
dry cold weather; while that from the north-east
to the south, is usually attended by clear, mild
weather. The south and south-west winds are
warm and oppressive. The westerly, or atlantic
winds, are the most prevalent; the north wind
blows feebly, and is not frequent; the oppressive
southerly winds are also infrequent, and seldom

continue beyond twenty-four hours. Indeed, Pau
appears to be almost exempt from the oppressive
southerly winds, on the one hand, and the cold
north-west winds on the other; both of which
prevail over this part of France generally. After
the west, the easterly winds are the most
frequent; and these, and the west usually, alternate: and it is observed that, according as the
one or the other prevails, the weather is rainy,
or dry and pleasant.

Though from the more frequent occurrence of
westerly winds, this climate may be said to be
rainy, still it is not subject to some of the evils
which commonly attend humid climates, or, at
least, it suffers from them in a less degree than
these generally do. Rain seldom continues above
two days at a time, and is usually followed in a
few hours by warm sunshine; while the ground,
from the absorbing nature of the soil, dries rapidly.
The atmosphere, generally speaking, is also remarkably free from moisture, as indicated by
the hygrometer. In October, some snow generally falls on the centre chain of the Pyrenees;
and, at Pau, this fall is marked by a sudden
change of temperature, the weather becoming
rainy and chilly. In November, the weather
clears up and becomes milder. December and
January are cold and dry; frost and slight snow-
showers then occur, but the snow does not lie
on the ground. The sun is bright and warm,

and from twelve till three o'clock an invalid may
generally take exercise. February is milder; but
towards the end of this month the spring rains
fall, and the weather is then chilly and disagreeable. March is mild, but variable, though there
are no cutting winds. In spring, westerly winds,
which are soft and mild, accompanied with rain,
alternate with dry easterly winds, also of a mild
character. Hence it is, that the vernal exacer-
bation of inflammatory affections of the stomach
and lungs, so commonly observed in other climates,
is little felt by invalids at Pau. Vegetation bursts
forth in the first week of April, which is a warm
month. May resembles April, but is warmer.
In June, the weather is hot and fine. July,
August and September, are very hot months, the
thermometer sometimes rising as high as 94° in
the shade, with a very powerful sun, preventing
exercise from eight in the morning till seven in
the evening.

According to Dr. Playfair, the good qualities
of Pau may be summed up as follows : Calmness,
moderate cold, bright sunshine of considerable
power even in winter, a dry state of atmosphere
and of the soil, and rains of short duration.
Against these must be placed—changeableness,
the fine weather being as short-lived as the bad ;
rapid variations of temperature, within moderate
limits however; and heavy rains in autumn and
spring.

Pau is upon the whole healthy. Measles, scarlatina, and hooping cough, are generally mild, and
croup almost unknown. Intermitting and bilious
fevers, and rheumatism, are the most prevalent
diseases. Rheumatism, according to a native
author, is the only disease that is very common;
it exists almost as an endemic, and stimulates
or complicates almost all the other diseases.*
Goitre is also very common among the peasantry.
The intermitting fevers occur chiefly among those
of the peasants who frequent the low damp
grounds in the neighbourhood. Scrofula is rare,
and consumption not a common disease.

There are several circumstances in the climate
of Pau which render it a favourable residence for
a certain class of invalids. The atmosphere, when
it does not rain, is dry, and the weather fine, and
there are neither fogs nor cold piercing winds.
The characteristic quality of the climate, however,
is the comparative mildness of its spring, and
exemption from cold cutting winds. While the
winter is 3° colder than the warmest parts of
England, and 6° colder than Rome, the *spring*
is 5½° warmer than the former, and only 2½°
colder than the latter. The mildness of the spring,
and its little liability to winds, render this place
favourable to chronic affections of the larynx,
trachea and bronchia. In gastric dyspepsia also,

* Journal de Physiologie, tom. vii., p. 203.

Dr. Playfair has found it beneficial, and he has seen it useful in a few cases of asthma.

Upon the whole, Pau appears to be one of the most desirable winter residences in the south-west part of France, for invalids labouring under chronic affections of the mucous membranes. In the same class of diseases, the mineral waters of the Pyrenees are also very beneficial; and it may be convenient, and adviseable, for the invalid who has derived benefit from a course of these waters, to pass the winter at Pau, with a view of returning to them in the following season. These waters may also be easily transported to Pau, and used occasionally during the winter. Those of *Bonnes,* which retain their qualities well, and are among the most efficacious of the waters of the Pyrenees, are at no great distance.

With delicate children, Dr. Playfair found the climate agree well, especially when they removed to the mountains during the summer.

Invalids labouring under, or liable to attacks of rheumatism, should, of course, avoid Pau. In bronchial diseases, also, when accompanied with much general relaxation of the system, and with copious expectoration and dyspnœa, the climate will not in general prove beneficial; and Dr. Playfair considers it too changeable in consumptive diseases.

Invalids who mean to pass the winter at Pau should arrive there in the end of September, or very early in October. In selecting apartments, (which are not very numerous,) they should recollect that it is of importance that these should have a southern aspect.

In fixing the period for leaving Pau, the destination of the person must be taken into account. If the object is to return to England, he may leave it in May; if he means to spend the summer among the Pyrenees, he should not leave it before June. The best season for using the mineral waters of the Pyrenees commences about the first of July.

SOUTH-EAST OF FRANCE.

Various places in the south-east of France have been, at different times, recommended as affording a good winter climate for consumptive patients; but nothing can be more unaccountable than how such an advice ever came to be given; as the experience of later years is in complete opposition to it, and the general and leading characters of the climate show, that there never was the least reason to sanction it. That the country which has always been infested by the terrible *Circius*, should have been chosen for the residence of the delicate and sensitive sufferer from pulmonary disease, is a striking proof of the very loose observations upon which medical opinions respecting climate have been formed. How this practice of sending consumptive invalids to the south-east of France, originated, it is not of importance to inquire; that it is founded on error, I think, I shall be able to prove, by a reference to the physical characters of the climate, the actual prevalence of consumption among the inhabitants, and, I may add, the total want of success which has attended the measure.

The mean annual temperature of *Provence* generally, is 58°; that is, about 7° warmer than the south-west of England, 3° warmer than the southwest of France, and about a degree below Italy, including the climate of the lower Apennines. Its *winter* temperature is 43°; being only $1\frac{1}{2}$° above the south-west of England, and 1° above the southwest of France, while it is 3° under Italy. The *spring* temperature is 55°; namely, 6° above the south-west of England, 1° above the south-west of France, and 2° below Italy. The temperature is distributed very unequally through the year; the difference of the mean of the warmest and the coldest months being 35°; this in the south-west of England is 22°, in the south-west of France 30°, in Italy 32°, and in Madeira only 14°.

Dryness is one of the most remarkable characters of the climate of Provence. At Marseilles and Toulon, about 19 inches of rain fall annually. This is less by six inches than what falls at London, and is not half so much as falls in the south-western extremity of Cornwall.

The annual number of days on which rain falls in Provence, is only 67, while at London it is 178. Again, in Provence (at Toulon) the quantity of water evaporated annually, is 40 inches, while at Paris it is 32 inches, at Gosport 25, and at London only 24. When these circumstances are taken into consideration, together with the high mean temperature of the place, Provence must appear the driest district of Europe. Indeed, the dry nature of the soil, and the bare parched aspect of the country, bespeak such a climate.

The general character of the climate of the South-East of France, therefore, is dry, hot, harsh, and irritating. Absolutely warmer than our own Island, and the south-western parts of France, its temperature is distributed through the year and through the day with great irregularity. It has a much wider range of temperature than our own climate; this being, when compared to that of England, as three to one for the year, and as two to one for the day. Sometimes the winter is very rigorous. In 1709, the ports of Marseilles and Toulon were frozen over; and, indeed, in ordinary years, the orange-trees are occasionally killed by the cold in the most sheltered parts of Provence. The temperature, no doubt, remains more steady from day to day than our own; but its changes, though less frequent, are more sudden and extensive.

This tract of country is subject also to keen,

cold northerly winds, especially the *mistral*, which prevails during the winter and spring, and is most injurious to pulmonary diseases.

Although decidedly improper for consumptive patients, and for those labouring under irritation of the mucous membranes of the digestive or pulmonary organs, more especially irritation of the stomach, larynx, or trachea, this climate may prove useful to invalids of a different class. On persons of a torpid, or relaxed habit of body, and of a gloomy, desponding cast of mind, with whom a moist relaxing atmosphere disagrees, the keen, bracing, dry air of Provence, and its brilliant skies, will often produce a beneficial effect. In some cases of chronic intermittent fevers also, it proves very favourable.

The distinctive characters of the climate we have been considering, prevail more or less in the different places resorted to by invalids, but none can be considered as exempt from them. The following is the order in which they ought to be preferred: *Hyères, Toulon, Marseilles, Montpelier, Aix, Nismes, Avignon.* The remarks which I have to make on these places individually, are derived partly from native practitioners, and partly from my own observation ; and it will be found, I think, that the particular facts very much confirm the general character given of the whole South-East of France, from Montpelier to Nice.

MONTPELIER.

The celebrity of the medical school of Montpelier had probably a considerable share in giving rise to the character which this place obtained for the benignity of its climate—*olim Cous nunc Monspeliensis.* But whatever may have been the merits of its medical school, it will be easy to show, that the climate little deserved the reputation which it long enjoyed, and, in some degree, still enjoys in England, as a residence for the consumptive. I prefer the evidence afforded on this subject by native authors. M. Murat, in his Medical Topography of Montpelier, published in 1810, states, on the authority of M. Fournier, the following proportion of deaths from consumption, at the Hotel Dieu, of that city, in the year 1763: The total number of patients that passed through this Hospital in the course of the year was 2,756. The total number of deaths was 154; and of this number 55 died of pulmonary consumption; that is, more than a third of the whole. After alluding to Mr. Fouquier's opinion, that phthisis was still more frequent at a former period, he adds, "Mais la phthisie pulmonaire n'est que trop répandue dans ce pays : elle y enlève même des familles entières ; et la position de la ville, et la constitution sèche et variable des saisons physiques, sont des causes locales qui la déveloperont toujours."* M. Fournier, the author from whom the above calculations are taken, observes, when noticing the prevalence of northerly winds at Montpelier, during the winter and spring, " Il faut avoir la poitrine bien bonne et bien constitutée pour résister a ses impressions."† Other circumstances in the topography and nature of the climate of Montpelier might be stated to show its unfitness as a residence for consumptive patients, but surely it is unnecessary to adduce further evidence on the subject.

MARSEILLES.

This place is but little intitled to claim any exemption from the general character of the climate of Provence. It is open to the full influence of the cold winds of this country, and especially to the mistral. When the weather does permit them to go out, there is, moreover, no part of the neighbourhood of Marseilles, where invalids can take exercise, one of the principal objects for which they left their own climate. The country around the city is divided into small properties, each enclosed by high walls, between which the roads in every direction lead for miles. The dry, arid nature of the soil, renders these roads in general

* Topographie Médicale de la Ville de Montpelier, p. 149.

† Recueil d' observations de Médecine des Hôpitaux Militaires par. M. Richard de Hautsierck, tom. II., p. 5.

very dusty, and their narrow winding form subjects them to gusts of wind; both of which circumstances make them most improper exercising ground, for invalids labouring under pulmonary irritation. Indeed, it may be almost said, that there is no country about Marseilles for the stranger residing there. But the character of the climate is still more objectionable. It is dry, variable, and subject to cold irritating winds, which are particularly injurious to consumptive patients. Marseilles is, indeed, one of the towns in France in which pulmonary consumption is most prevalent. A large proportion of the youth of both sexes is carried off by it. Females, from fourteen to eighteen years of age, are said to be its most frequent victims. To use the words of a native author: " Il fait des ravages inouiés en moissonnant la plus belle jeunesse. " * Scrofula attacking the external parts of the body, is rather a rare occurrence at Marseilles. Pleurisy and catarrh are frequent ; as are cancer and cutaneous eruptions. Diseases of the uterine system are also common.

Invalids requiring a dry climate, and capable of bearing keen, cold winds, will be benefited by a residence at Marseilles : Patients labouring under intermittent fevers often get rid of them without medicine, on coming to this place.

* Exposé des travaux de la Societé de Médecine de Marseille, 1816, par M. Sigaud, p. 14.

AIX.

Aix, is another place which, for a time, enjoyed a degree of reputation in England as a winter residence for the consumptive; though with no more reason than the places we have just mentioned. The mean annual temperature of Aix is 56°, about 4° below that of Marseilles; and its extreme annual range of temperature is no less than 83°, viz., ten degrees more than that of Marseilles. Its situation exposes it, in a particular manner, to the mistral and other cold winds. The inhabitants are, in consequence, very subject to pulmonary complaints. "L' atmosphére d' Aix," says the author of the natural history of Provence, "est souvent agitée par le souffle des vents qui s'y font sentir plus qu'ailleurs." To these winds, he says are owing "des rheums frequens, des fièvres catarrhales, des maladies de poitrine et des rheumatismes." He further adds,—" Il n'y a point des maladies endemiques; la *phthisie* paroit y faire seulement quelque ravage parmi le peuple. On voit tres peu de veillards au dela de 75 ans. La vie moyenne des hommes ne s'etend pas au dessus de 30 ans. " *

* Histoire naturelle de la Provence. par M. Darluc, M. D. Avignon, 1782. Tom. I., p. 15, &c.

HYERES.

The little town of Hyères, agreeably situated on
the southern declivity of a hill, about two miles
from the shores of the Mediterranean, and twelve
from Toulon, is the least exceptionable residence
for the pulmonary invalid in Provence. It is in
some degree protected from the northerly winds,
and has the advantage of being situated in a
beautiful, open country. Immediately under the
town the orange-tree (of the hardiest species, however) is cultivated in abundance. It thrives very
well, and, in general, is little injured by the winter.
It has, nevertheless, happened several times,
although after an interval of many years, that the
cold has been sufficiently intense to destroy the
whole orange-trees at Hyères in one night. This
occurred last in the winter of 1820, on which
occasion a single orange-tree did not escape; and
many of the olive-trees, in the most exposed
situations, were also partially killed.

The lower grounds are occupied with vines and
corn, and about the basis of the hills the olive is
extensively cultivated, and attains a considerable
size. The hills immediately surrounding Hyères
are finely covered with evergreen shrubs, affording
a striking contrast to the bare, unseemly aspect,
which the hills of Provence generally present.

G

The thyme, rosemary, lavender, and many other aromatic plants, grow here in abundance; and several of these we found blooming in December. With all these indications of mildness, Hyères is by no means sufficiently protected from the mistral, to render it a desirable residence for consumptive invalids, (setting aside other objections from the nature of the climate,) although it has been strongly recommended as such. It is true that about the base of the hills there are some spots sheltered from the mistral, where the invalid might enjoy several hours in the open air almost every day; but the difficulty is to reach them at the time they would be most useful. The chilly blast sweeping round every exposed corner forbids the valetudinarian venturing there, except in a close carriage, while the roads leading to these places do not admit wheeled vehicles. When the weather does permit, the invalid residing at Hyères may enjoy the advantage of a variety of rides through a fine open country. But when the mistral blows with any degree of force, he will require to keep the house, if his chest is delicate; and he must even be cautious of exposing himself to the milder degrees of this wind, which, independent of its low temperature, is very irritating. With all these objections, the climate of Hyères is the mildest in Provence. And the invalid may feel assured, that whatever inconveniences he is subjected to from the cold winds at this place, he would have experienced more severely in any other part of the south-eastern district.

Hyères is not subject to any particular diseases. The marshy ground below the town, which formerly gave rise to intermittent fevers during the summer and autumn, has been pretty well drained. I was informed by the resident medical men that pulmonary consumption is not frequent: a circumstance which they bring forward as a proof of the salubrity of the place. This comparative exemption from consumption (if it really exist) may, in some measure, depend on the inhabitants being employed chiefly in the labours of the field; for the soil is principally cultivated by manual labour. This little town is so confined and limited, that it affords little choice of situation.

NICE.

The climate of Nice approximates more nearly in its general characters to that of Provence, which has just been described, than to any other. Its mean annual temperature is 59°, being 9° warmer than London, 7° warmer than Penzance, 1° colder than Rome, and 5° colder than Madeira. The mean temperature of *winter* is 48°; that is, nearly 9° warmer than London, 4° warmer than Penzance, 1° colder than Rome, and 12° colder than Madeira. The mean temperature of *spring* is 56°; being 7°

warmer than London, 6° warmer than Penzance, 1° colder than Rome, and 6° colder than Madeira. The temperature throughout the year is more equally distributed at Nice than at any place in the South of Europe, of which we have accounts, except Rome and Cadiz; the difference of the warmest and coldest months being only 28°, and the mean difference of successive months only 4°.74.

The range of temperature for the day is also less at Nice than at any part of the South of Europe; and in steadiness of temperature it ranks next to Madeira.

The weather at Nice during the winter is comparatively settled and fine, the atmosphere being generally clear, and the sky remarkable for its brilliancy. The temperature seldom sinks to. the freezing point, and when it does, it is only during the night; so that vegetation is never altogether suspended. Indeed, at Nice, winter is a season of flowers, the dryness of the air rendering the same degree of cold less injurious to them, than it would be in a more humid atmosphere. The mild and equable character of the climate of Nice depends in a great measure on its position, with respect to the neighbouring mountains and the sea. The maritime Alps rise immediately behind it, and form a lofty barrier which shelters it from the northerly winds during winter; while, on the other hand, the heat during summer is moderated by the cool sea-breeze, which prevails here every day, with a regularity almost equal to that of a tropical climate. "Cet alizé mediterraneen," says M. Risso, "toujours doux, frais et tranquille, s' eleve periodiquement vers neuf à dix heures du matin, cesse souvent vers les quatre heures après midi, et s' étend dans l'interieur de nos Alpes rarement au delà de huit myriamètres.* " These circumstances explain the small annual range of temperature at this place, already noticed, and which a reference to the table in the appendix will show to be much less than at most parts of Italy.

Notwithstanding the extent, however, to which Nice and its environs are encircled by mountains, (and it is so in a great measure from W. S. W., to E. S. E.,) it is by no means exempt from cold winds during the winter, and still less so during the spring. The easterly winds are the most prevalent during the latter season. They range from east to north-east, frequently blow with considerable force, and are often accompanied with a hazy, cloudy state of atmosphere. Sometimes this wind sets in towards the forenoon, at other times not until the afternoon. When the early part of the day is fine, it never

---

* Histoire Naturelle des Principales Productions de l'Europe Meridionale, et particulièrement de celles des Environs de Nice. 1826. par A. Risso. Vol. I., p. 219.

To this excellent work I beg leave to refer my readers who may be desirous of information respecting the Natural History of the South of Europe.

should be lost for exercise ; as the afternoon frequently proves cold and windy, after a calm, mild,
morning.

From the north-west, or mistral, which is the
scourge of Provence, Nice is pretty well sheltered.
The force of this wind seems to be broken, and
directed to the southward by the Estrelles, a chain
of mountains between Frejus and Cannes. But,
although the mistral is never experienced in its full
power at Nice, or only towards its termination,
when it takes a more westerly direction, (*la queue
de la Mistral,* as it is called,) the keen, dry quality
of the air is very sensibly felt whilst it prevails.
It sets in generally about two or three o'clock
in the afternoon, and is not of long duration. It
seldom blows strong directly from the north,
though the air is very sharp when the wind is in
that quarter. The northerly gales appear to pass
obliquely over Nice.* The sirocco rarely blows,
and when it does, it is gentle, and not unpleasant
to the feelings of invalids in general. But the
sharp, chilling, easterly winds are the greatest

* "On éprouve fort rarement," says M. Risso, "tout sa force
dans les couches inférieures de l'air qui environnent le plateau de
Nice, à cause du triple rang de montagnes qui l'entourent; il
occupe presque toujours les couches supérieurs, et descend en
pente comme un grand torrent aerien sur la mer; car on aperçoit
a un kilomètre du rivage qu' il commence à en friser la surface
pour former un peu plus loin des vagues qui, s'élévant les unes
sur les autres, vont porter les tempêtes sur les côtes boréales
d' Afrique. *Hist. Nat.,*Vol. I., p. 216.

enemy the invalid has to contend with at this place; and the prevalence of these during the months of March and April is admitted, I believe, by all who have felt them, to form a great objection to this climate, especially in pulmonary diseases.

The climate of Nice is altogether a very dry one. Rain falls chiefly during particular seasons. From the middle of October to the middle of November it generally rains a good deal; also about the winter solstice there is commonly some rain, and again, after the vernal equinox. The quantity of rain that falls during the year has not been accurately estimated.

Upon the whole, in the physical qualities of its climate, Nice possesses some advantages over the neighbouring countries of Provence and Italy, inasmuch as it may be said to be free from the sirocco of the latter, and protected from the mistral of the former.

Nice is a healthy place. It is exempt from endemic diseases, and epidemics are said to be rare. Catarrhal affections and inflammation of the lungs rank among the most frequent diseases. The latter is especially common and violent in the spring, and is generally complicated with irritation of the digestive organs. Pulmonary consumption, though much less frequent than in England and France, still carries off a certain proportion of the inhabitants, especially in the

town. The proportion of deaths in the hospital
from this disease, is said to be about one-seventh
of the whole mortality. Gastric fever and chronic
gastritis are very common diseases. Indeed,
gastric irritation appears to be the prevailing
endemic disorder of the place; and hence almost
all other diseases are complicated with more or
less of it. Intermittent fevers are not unfrequent
among the peasantry living or labouring in unhealthy situations. The flat ground on the banks of
the Var is, of all situations in the vicinity, the most
fruitful source of these fevers. The guard stationed
on the bridge which crosses this boundary stream
are frequently attacked with agues, during the
unhealthy season, though they remain there only a
few days at a time. This is a disease, however,
from which the winter resident at Nice has nothing
to fear. Dr. Skirving, during a long residence there,
has only met with one case of ague amongst the
strangers. Diseases of the eyes are very prevalent,
particularly amaurosis and cataract ; cutaneous
diseases are also very common. The elephantiasis
of the Greeks is occasionally found in certain warm
spots in the neighbourhood. It is also found
sometimes in the vicinity of Marseilles, and, I
believe, along the whole of this coast. I think it
is less common in Italy, except perhaps at Naples.

In proceeding to describe the effects of the
climate of Nice on disease, I feel it due to Dr.

Skirving, who has practised there many years, to state, that I am much indebted to him for favouring me with the results of his extensive experience.

In *Consumption*, the disease with which the climate of Nice has been chiefly associated in the minds of medical men in this country, little benefit I fear is to be expected. When this disease is complicated with an inflammatory, or highly irritable state of the mucous membranes of the larynx, trachea, or bronchia, or of the stomach, Nice is decidedly an unfavourable climate; and, without extreme care on the part of such patients, and a very strict regimen, the complaint will in all probability be aggravated by a residence here. Indeed, the cases of consumption which ought to be sent to Nice are of rare occurrence. If there are any such, it is when the disease exists in torpid habits, of little susceptibility, or not much disposed to irritation; and when it is free from the complications which have been just mentioned. Even the propriety of selecting Nice as a residence for persons merely threatened with consumption, will depend much upon the constitution of the individual. Dr. Skirving has met with cases which leave no doubt on his mind, that a residence for one or two winters often proves of advantage, as a preventive measure, in young persons threatened with this disease; and even in some cases when there was every reason to believe that tubercles already existed in the lungs, the climate has appeared to be useful. But in the advanced stage of consumption, his opinion, founded on eight years' experience, accords with what has been already stated; and this is still further supported by the testimony of Professor Fodere, of Strasbourg, who resided six years at Nice.* Indeed, sending consumptive patients in this stage to Nice, will in a great majority of cases prove more injurious than beneficial.

In *Chronic Bronchial* diseases, which often simulate phthisis, very salutary effects are produced by a residence at this place. Such patients generally pass the winter with little comparative suffering from their complaint, and with benefit to their general health. They are here able to be much in the open air, whereas if they had remained in England, they would in all probability have been confined during the greater part of the winter to the house. The particular kind of bronchial disease most benefited by a residence at Nice, is that accompanied with copious expectoration, whether complicated with asthma *(humoral asthma)* or otherwise; and in the chronic catarrh of aged people it is particularly beneficial. This variety of bronchial disease is directly the reverse of that which is benefited by the south-west of France and

---

* See Voyage aux Alpes Maritimes, ou Histoire Naturelle, agraire, civile et médicale du pays de Nice, &c., Strasbourg, 1823.

of England: and I think it important here to remark, that unless the distinctions which I have pointed out in bronchial diseases, and their complications, are attended to, great errors must be committed in selecting a residence for such patients. But for fuller information on this subject, I must refer the reader to the article on " Bronchial Diseases."

Of pure *Nervous Asthma,* neither Dr. Skirving nor myself have seen a sufficient number of cases to enable us to come to any satisfactory conclusion on the effect of this climate on that disease. Some cases of asthma, complicated with diseases of the heart, have certainly benefited by a winter's residence here.

The *gouty* invalid may in most cases escape his usual winter attack at this place, and, provided he lives with prudence, he may afterwards return to his own country with improved health.

In *Chronic Rheumatism,* the climate is generally very beneficial; and its advantages are also remarkable in *Scrofulous Complaints.* On children with enlarged lymphatic glands, and even with symptoms indicative of incipient mesenteric disease, the climate exerts a very favourable influence. Indeed, with children in general, it agrees remarkably well.

In what is commonly called dyspeptic complaints, and the numerous train of hypochondriacal and nervous symptoms which often originate in such a source, Nice is beneficial. But here, again, it is necessary to distinguish the particular character of the affection. The cases of dyspepsia most benefited, are those accompanied with a torpid, relaxed state of the system, with little epigastric tenderness, or any of those symptoms which denote an inflamed or very irritable state of the mucous membrane of the stomach. Where the latter state is the cause of the dyspeptic symptoms, Nice will decidedly disagree ; indeed, as I have already observed, a degree of this affection is almost endemic there. But I must refer to the article on " Disorders of the Digestive Organs" for more precise directions regarding the best winter residence for persons suffering from stomach complaints.

In all cases where there is great relaxation and torpor of the constitution, the climate of Nice is extremely useful. In young females labouring under such a state of system, connected with irregularities of the uterine functions, either when these have not been established at the usual period, or when they have afterwards been suppressed, marked benefit may generally be expected. In indicating the class of cases alluded to, as likely to be benefited by the climate of Nice, I would designate them to the practical physician as those that are usually relieved by chalybeates.

In a numerous class of patients, whose constitutions have been injured by a long residence in tropical countries, by mercury, &c., and in which a dry and rather exciting climate is indicated, Nice will prove favourable. Some cases of chronic paralysis, not connected with cerebral disease, have also been found to derive considerable benefit from a residence at this place.

In stating its general influence on the animal œconomy, I would say—that the climate of Nice is warm, exhilirating, and exciting, but upon the whole, irritating,—at least to highly sensitive constitutions. It is extremely favourable to the productions of the vegetable kingdom, some of which flourish here in a degree of luxuriance that is scarcely to be equalled in the other parts of the south of Europe.*

Invalids who pass the winter at Nice, scarcely ever reside in the town. Some good lodgings, and tolerably well situated, overlooking the terrace,

---

* " Peu de contrées méridionales de l'Europe offrent un tableau aussi varié en vegetaux indigènes et exotiques que les environs de Nice. Dans le fond, c'est une masse d'oliviers qui s'étend sur toutes les collines, et disparaît insensiblement à mesure qu'elle s'eloigne du rivage de la mer. Sur le devant, ce sont des orangers, des bigaradiers, des limoniers, disposés en jardins qui offrent toute la luxe des Hespérides. Pour relever la sombre verdure des uns et la monotonie des autres, des caroubiers, des figuiers, des jujubiers, des raquettiers, des dattiers, des grenadiers, et toutes sortes d'arbres fruitiers distribués sans ordre, en étalant toute leur vigueur, achèvent d'orner etd 'embellir ce bel ensemble."—*Histoire Naturelle*, &c., Vol. I., p. 313, &c.

are, however, now to be had; but in the
suburb, called the *Croix de Marbre,* and along
the sea-beach, from the town to the ridge of
mountains which bounds the plain on the west,
the largest and best houses are to be found; and
here strangers generally reside. At the foot of
the hill on which stood *Cimiez,* there are also
some good houses; and this is a situation preferable to the lower part of the plain for patients
very susceptible of injury from damp.

Invalids should endeavour to arrive at Nice
about the middle of October, or sooner, and
should not leave it before the beginning of May.
Whatever inconvenience they may here suffer
from the spring winds, they will experience in a
greater degree by returning through the South
of France; and, accordingly, both Dr. Skirving
and myself have known invalids suffer materially
from the winds of Provence by leaving Nice too
early. It is true that the new road which has
lately been opened between Nice and Genoa,
admits of the invalid moving in that direction,
at a much earlier period than it would be adviseable for him to return over the Estrelles to
Provence; and when the climate of Nice is found
to disagree, a change in the spring in the direction
of Genoa may, in some cases, be adviseable.

VILLA FRANCA.

Immediately to the eastward of Montalbano, which separates the bay of Villa Franca from that of Nice, is situated this little town. It stands at the bottom of a beautiful small bay, or harbour, and on the base, or rather declivity of a steep and lofty ridge of mountains, which rise immediately behind it. From the north and north-west winds, this place is certainly more effectually protected than Nice, but, on the other hand, it is open to the whole range of easterly winds, which we have seen to be the most prevalent of the spring winds, and the most injurious to the invalid. The climate of Villa Franca, though somewhat drier and warmer than that of Nice, has really no essential superiority over it, and, moreover, there are very few accommodations for invalids. MENTON is also a very sheltered spot, about fourteen miles from Nice on the Genoa road; and SAN REMO, still further, is even more protected from easterly winds. The great mildness of both places is indicated by the flourishing state of their lemon plantations. And at Bordighera, in the neighbourhood of the latter, the palm-tree is cultivated on a large scale for the sake of its etiolated leaves, of which it has long afforded a supply for the ceremonies of the church of

Rome. But the want of accommodation at these places, at present, prevents the invalid, to whom a change from Nice might be advantageous, from availing himself of it. The increased number of travellers, however, who will in future pass by the new road, now open from Nice to Genoa, will most probably soon afford the means of improving the accommodation along this beautiful coast.

ITALY.

Italy possesses great diversity of climate, but my observations are limited to that tract which is situated between the northern shores of the Mediterranean, and the southern base of the Apennines. The climate which prevails over the whole of this region, while it exhibits a great similarity of character, differs in several respects from any of the climates already noticed: it is considerably warmer and less humid, but subject to a greater range of temperature, than that of the south-west of France; it is softer, less dry, and less harsh and irritating than that of Provence; suffering more from the heavy oppressive winds of the south, and less from the dry searching winds of the north.

The principal circumstance which appears to modify the general character of this climate at the different places, is, their relative position with respect to the sea-shore and the Apennines. In this there is some variety: Genoa and Naples are in the vicinity of both, as the mountains at these places approach closely to the Mediterranean;

Pisa is only a few miles distant from the latter, and close to the Tusean hills, which are a branch of the lower Apennines; Rome is about twelve miles from the coast, and nearly twice that distance from the mountains; Florence is quite inland, and so embosomed in the Apennines, as to have the character of its climate thereby very materially affected—to such a degree, indeed, as scarcely to admit of its being classed with the other Italian climates.

GENOA.

The situation of Genoa, hemmed in between a range of steep mountains and the sea, with little or no surrounding country well adapted for exercise, renders it an unsuitable residence for invalids generally : nor is there much in the character of the climate to recommend it. The summer is hotter, and the winter colder than at Nice; the difference between the mean temperature of the warmest and coldest months being 35°. The distribution of heat through the year is also very unequal, and the temperature by no means steady from day to day. The air is sharp and exciting, but with less of the irritating quality than that of the south-east of France. The climate is, on the whole, dry and healthy, but not suitable to delicate, sensitive invalids. It is more congenial to relaxed, phlegmatic habits. Dys-

peptic complaints and gout are said to prevail
less at Genoa than at most parts of Italy ; and
I have certainly known gouty patients find themselves more comfortable, and have fewer and less
severe paroxysms here, than either in the south
of France or other parts of Italy. For pulmonary
affections, Genoa is decidedly an improper residence. It is subject to frequent and rapid changes
of temperature, and to dry, cold winds from the
north, alternating with warm, humid winds from
the south-east,—the two prevailing winds of the
place. To these rapid changes are attributed the
inflammatory affections of the respiratory organs,
which, with tubercular consumption, cause the
greater part of the mortality of Genoa. In some
places in the neighbourhood, more sheltered from
these winds, inflammatory affections of the lungs
are much less common than in the city and its
immediate vicinity. Consumption is said to be
less rapid in its course at Genoa than in Provence.
Rheumatism is frequent, while gout, as already
mentioned, is comparatively a rare disease. Dysentery generally prevails a good deal during the
summer months. Scrofula is common. Intermittent fevers are rare, and of mild character.
Nervous affections are also comparatively rare,
and so are calculous diseases. The healthiest
months in the year are April, May, June, September, and October ; the more unhealthy are
December, January, February, and August.

FLORENCE.

Though Florence is one of the most agreeable residences in Italy, it is far fron being a favourable climate for an invalid, and, least of all, for an invalid disposed to consumption.

Its situation among the lower Apennines, by which it is almost encircled, and the summits of which are covered with snow during the winter, together with its full exposure to the current of the valley of the Arno, renders Florence subject to sudden transitions of temperature, and to cold piercing winds during the winter and spring. Fogs, too, are more common here than at most parts of southern Italy. The winter temperature is upon the whole low, while that of the summer is high. The mean annual temperature is only $1\frac{1}{2}°$ below that of Rome; but this is owing to the great heat of summer at Florence; for the winter is only $4°$ warmer than that of London, and is nearly of the same temperature as the winter at Penzance. The difference between the mean temperature of the warmest and coldest months is $36°$, which is one degree more than that of Provence. Nevertheless, although the daily, monthly, and annual range of temperature are very great, the climate is not more variable or unsteady from day to day than that of Rome, and is less so than that of Naples. The annual range of atmospheric pressure is greater than that of the neighbouring places. The annual fall of rain at Florence is 31. 6 inches, but the number of days on which rain falls is only 103, being fewer than at Rome. In the winter the air is·rather chilly, and loaded with moisture.

I do not know any class of invalids for whom Florence offers an adviseable residence. My own opinion, founded partly on observation, and partly on the reports of invalids, perfectly accords with that of Dr. Seymour of London, and Dr. Down of Southampton, whose more extensive opportunities of observation during a long residence and extensive practice at Florence, make their testimony of greater value. " The winter," says Dr. Down, " is extremely severe and wet, and the spring changeable, consequently highly injurious in complaints of the chest. The inhabitants are very subject to diseases of the lungs; and the acute inflammation of this organ, known under the popular name of *Mal di petto*, carries off yearly in the winter and spring an amazing number of them, particularly of the poorer classes, whose houses are ill calculated to afford protection against the cold and rains of these seasons."* Florence is one of the places in Italy which agrees least with children. Intestinal worms are particularly common there, and dysentery is pre-

---

* Observations on the Nature and Treatment of Fevers and Bowel Complaints, &c., in Greece, by J. Somers Down, M. D.

valent in autumn. Pellagra, a disease almost peculiar to Lombardy, is endemic in some parts of the neighbouring vallies of the Apennines.

Florence itself is not subject to any endemic disease; and to persons not likely to suffer from the vicissitudes of temperature, which have been noticed, and who can support the great heat of summer, it holds out many inducements as a residence during the whole year.

PISA.

Pisa has long had the reputation of being one of the mildest and most favourable climates in Italy for consumptive patients. It has accordingly been frequented, and continues to be so, by invalids from this country. It is even resorted to, during the winter, by invalids from the rest of Tuscany, from the neighbouring states of Lucca, and occasionally, also, from Lombardy.

The town is built on the banks of the Arno, about five miles from the sea-shore. The surrounding country is flat, except towards the north, where there is a range of hills, which shelter it in some measure from the winds of that quarter. It is also protected in a considerable degree from easterly winds by the lower Tuscan hills. In flowing through Pisa, the Arno makes a semi-circular sweep to the north, so that the buildings on the northern bank of the river (*Lung' Arno*) assume the form of a crescent facing the south, and shelter the greater part of the broad space between them and the river from northerly winds. This is the principal, and certainly the best residence for delicate invalids.

Pisa is not so warm as Rome in winter, and is hotter in summer. In *winter* it is 7° warmer than London, and 2° warmer than Penzance. In *spring* it is 8° warmer than London, and about 7° warmer than Penzance. The range of temperature between day and night is very considerable. According to Professor Piazzini, the fall of rain annually is very great, being 45.66 inches, which is nearly as much as falls in Cornwall. The climate of Pisa is genial, but rather heavy and damp. It is softer than that of Nice, but not so warm ; less soft, but less heavy and depressing than that of Rome. For invalids who are almost confined to the house, or whose power of taking exercise is much limited, Pisa offers advantages over either Rome or Nice : The Lung' Arno affords a warm site for their residence, as well as a sheltered terrace for their walks. But they must be careful to confine themselves to it. They should not venture into the cross streets before April.

The most common acute diseases are peripneumony, *(mal di petto,)* dysentery, and gastric fevers. Cataract and ophthalmia are common ; but this is the case over the whole southern parts of Italy. Phthisis pulmonalis is not a common disease, but chronic bronchial affections are frequent; and croup is occasionally met with. At one period, intermitting fevers were very prevalent about Pisa; but since the surrounding country has been drained and cultivated, they are comparatively rare. In the hospital, however, the double tertian is endemic; and a large proportion of the patients who undergo operations, have an attack of this fever, which sometimes even assumes the pernicious form.* Hospital gangrene is certainly more common in the hospital at Pisa than in most other hospitals in Italy. Nervous diseases likewise prevail, but not so much as at Rome. Affections of the bones appear to be more common here than usual, particularly that called spina ventosa. Calculous diseases are so rare, that Vacca, during thirty-two years that he had been operating on such patients from all parts of Italy, has not had occasion to operate on one Pisan.

---

* During my last visit to Pisa, the late Professor Vacca informed me that intermittent fevers were now so rare, that wishing to try the Piperine, a considerable time elapsed before they could find a case for the experiment. While he was studying at Pisa, the wards in summer had an additional row of beds on account of the number of intermittents. At that period there was a good deal of uncultivated land and stagnant water around the town.

NAPLES.

In its general characters the climate of Naples resembles that of Nice more than any other. As at Nice, the autumn and winter are generally mild, and the spring subject to cold, sharp, irritating winds, rendered more trying and hurtful to invalids, by the heat of a powerful sun. The climate of Naples is much more changeable than that of Nice; and, if somewhat softer in the winter, it is more damp and wet. The sirocco which is severely felt at Naples is little known at Nice. The mean annual temperature is higher than that of Rome, Pisa, or Nice; but the annual range of mean temperature is very corsiderable—being 30°; whilst that of Nice is but 28°; and that of Rome only 26°. The distribution of temperature in the different months is more unequal than at Nice or Rome. The daily range of temperature is also very great, being 2° more than at Rome. The temperature likewise varies very much from day to day, as will appear from the following statement :— The mean variation of successive days at Naples is 3°.36; at Rome it is 2°.80; at Leghorn 2°.44; at Nice 2°.33. The annual range of atmospheric pressure is very small,—somewhat less than at Rome, and very considerably less than in the south-east of France. Rain falls less frequently at Naples than at Rome.

Of the diseases of the inhabitants of Naples, catarrhal affections are the most frequent. Consumption is not very frequent, nor in general rapid in its course : autumn is said to be the most fatal season to the consumptive. Rheumatism is very frequent. Nervous affections are also common, as are cutaneous diseases, and diseases of the uterine system. Naples is not subject to any endemic disease, although intermittent fever is not unfrequent in some places in the outskirts of the city. Inflammation of the eyes appears very prevalent.

Of Naples as a residence for invalids it is unnecessary to say much. Consumptive patients should certainly not be sent there. The circumstances which have been pointed out in its climate, sufficiently mark it as a very unsuitable residence for this class of persons; and to the list of its defects must be added that of its topographical position, which affords no proper places for exercise, without such exposure as would prove highly injurious to delicate invalids. For chronic rheumatism it is, as compared with Nice and Rome, certainly inferior. Naples is however well suited as a winter residence for those who are labouring under general debility and derangement of the constitution without any marked local disease. The beauty of its situation, the brilliancy of its skies, and the interest excited by the surrounding scenery, render it a very desirable and very delightful winter residence, for those who rather require mental amusement and recreation for the restoration of their general health, than medical treatment for any particular disease.

With respect to choice of situation in Naples, invalids with whom a warm and rather close atmosphere agrees, will find themselves best in the *Chiája, Vittoria,* or *Chiatamone.* With patients labouring under nervous dyspepsia and nervous invalids generally, these places will not agree. The *Largo del Castello, Pizzo Falcone, San Lucia,* and *Largo del Vasto* afford more favourable residences for them.

The Neapolitan physicians generally condemn the vicinity of the sea in consumptive cases, and think such patients do better in the more sheltered places behind the town and in the neighbourhood of the *Studio;* but here strangers do not reside. Of the situations frequented by strangers, the Chiaja and Chiatamone afford altogether the best residences for pulmonary invalids. These situations are fully exposed to the south, and pretty well sheltered from the north; while their immediate vicinity to the public gardens (*Villa Reale*) is convenient for walking exercise. But, as I have already observed, Naples is altogether an unsuitable residence for pulmonary invalids.

I shall again have occasion to notice the climate of Naples when treating of a summer residence in Italy.

ROME.

The character of the climate of Rome is mild and soft, but rather relaxing and oppressive. Its mean annual temperature is 10° higher than that of London, 8° higher than Penzance, 6° higher than Pau, about 1° higher than Marseilles, Toulon, and Nice; 1° below that of Naples, and 4° below that of Madeira. The mean temperature of *winter* still remains 10° higher than that of London, but it is only 5° higher than Penzance; it is 7° higher than Pau, 1° higher than Nice, and somewhat higher than Naples; it is 4° colder than Cadiz, and 11° colder than Madeira. In *spring*, the mean temperature of Rome is 9° above London, 8° above Penzance, not quite 3° above Pau, and 1° above Nice and Provence; it is 1° colder than Naples, and only a little more than 4° colder than Madeira.

In *range* of temperature (the extent of which is the leading fault of the climate of the South of Europe) Rome has the advantage of Naples, Pisa, and Provence, but not of Nice. Its diurnal range is nearly double that of London, Gosport, Penzance, and Madeira. In steadiness of temperature from day to day, in which our own country, with the exception of Penzance, is so remarkably deficient, Rome follows Madeira, Nice,

Pisa, Leghorn, and the south-west of Cornwall,
but preceeds Naples and Pau.

With regard to humidity, Rome, though a soft,
cannot be considered a damp climate. Upon comparing it with the dry, parching climate of Provence,
and with that of Nice, we find that about one-third
more rain falls, and on a greater number of days
(117.) It is, however, considerably drier than
Pisa, and very much drier than the South-West of
France.

At Penzance there falls about one-third more
rain than at Rome, and the number of rainy days
is also about one-third greater. This circumstance,
together with the greater evaporation going on at
Rome, owing to its higher temperature, must make
a considerable difference in the hygrometrical state
of the atmosphere, at the two places. Rome is not
so dry as Madeira; as there falls one-sixth more
rain at the former place, and the proportion of wet
days is as 117 to 73. From these comparisons, it
would appear that the climate of Rome, in regard
to its physical qualities, is altogether the best of
any in Italy. One peculiarity of it, deserving
notice, is the stillness of its atmosphere; high
winds being comparatively of rare occurrence.
And this quality of calmness is valuable in a winter
climate for pulmonary diseases; more especially
for diseases of the larnyx, trachea and bronchia.
It is also of great importance to invalids generally,

as it enables them to take exercise in the open air at a much lower temperature, than they could otherwise do. To patients labouring under bronchial irritation, wind is peculiarly hurtful. When wind does occur at Rome, during the winter and spring, it is generally from the north, (tramontana,) at least when it continues for any considerable time. From this quarter there are occasional storms of cold wind; but these are of short duration, being limited, with surprizing regularity, to three days. The Tramontana is a dry, keen, and irritating wind, resembling in its effects the cold, sharp winds of Provence; and is equally to be guarded against by invalids; who should not stir out of the house while it blows with much force. The effects of this wind are accurately described by Celsus: "Aquilo tussim movet, fauces exasperat, ventrem adstringit, urinam supprimit, horrores excitat item dolorem lateris et pectoris. Sanum tamen corpus spissat et mobilius atque expeditius reddit.* " The southerly winds during the winter and spring do not produce much inconvenience to invalids at Rome. Even the relaxing and enervating effects of the *Sirocco* are not much felt, except by the more sensitive, and plethoric among the healthy, and by them only after it has continued to blow for a few days.

* Liber II., Cap. I.

Debilitated invalids, on the other hand, who suffer from great irritability, and a degree of morbid sensibility of body, commonly feel the winter sirocco pleasant. In its effects on the body this wind is directly opposed to the Tramontana. "Auster aures hebetat, sensus tardat, capitis dolorem movet, alvum solvit, totum corpus efficit hebes, humidum, languidum." * Notwithstanding the character given of this wind by Celsus, it is the favourite of the modern Romans; and during the prevalence of the winter sirocco they feel the full enjoyment of health. In the months of March and April, winds are more frequent at Rome; they set in generally in the forenoon, and continue till sunset, when they generally subside, leaving the nights calm and serene; and with a cloudless brilliancy which, at this season, is peculiar to Italy. The effects of these keen spring winds, combined with that of a powerful sun, are severely felt by the sensitive invalid; though, as far as I could observe or learn from the testimony of others, these effects are considerably less in degree than those resulting from the same causes, during this season, at Nice, and perhaps even at Pisa.

DISEASES.—Among the more prevalent diseases of Rome, *Malaria* fevers are the most remarkable; and, as the great endemic of the country, claim

* Celsus, loc. citat.

our first notice. The subject of Malaria has lately excited much attention in England; its effects having been more generally felt during the last few years than for a long period before. Although the subject is one of great interest, a formal or scientific disquisition on it, would be quite foreign to the object of this work. In the few remarks I am about to make, I shall, therefore, confine myself chiefly to those circumstances respecting Malaria, which it is important for travellers to know, with the view of enabling them to avoid its effects.

In the first place, I may observe, that the malaria fevers of Rome are exactly of the same nature, both in their origin and general characters, as the fevers which are so common in the fens of Lincolnshire and Essex, in our own country, in Holland, and in certain districts, I believe, over the whole globe; though the term malaria, which was for a certain time restricted to the fevers of Rome, but which has now become almost a generic name for these diseases, has given rise to some confusion on the subject, even among medical men. The form and aspect under which these fevers appear, may differ according to the concentration of the cause, or to some peculiar circumstances in the nature of the climate or season in which they occur; but it is the same disease, from the fens of Lincolnshire and the swamps of Walcheren, to the pestilential shores of Africa; only increased in severity, cæteris paribus, as the temperature of the climate increases. In England, and in Holland, these fevers generally appear in the simple intermitting form; often, but more rarely, in the remitting form; and they are, for the most part, easy of cure. In France, especially towards the south, the same fevers often assume a more formidable character. Those which from their unusual severity, and the peculiar character of their symptoms, have received the name of *Pernicious,* are by no means uncommon in the south-west of France; and in the rice districts of Lombardy, they are met with in all their varieties; and with a degree of severity, perhaps equal to the more aggravated forms of the malaria fevers of Rome.

These fevers have generally been attributed to the direct action of something exhaled from the soil; but of the nature of this agent we are quite ignorant, and its existence is even doubted by many. It is singular that this opinion, which originated with Lancisi, should be wearing away in Italy, whilst it may be said to be extending itself in England. By several Italian writers the disease has been attributed to the influence of sudden alternations of temperature, humidity of the atmosphere, and irregularities in living, &c.*

---

* See Richerche intorno alla causa della Febbre Perniciosa dominante nello Stato Romano, del Dr. Santarelli; also, Brevi Considerazioni, &c., by Prof. Folchi, of Rome, being a reply to an article on this subject in the Ed. Rev. Giorn. Arcad. T. xvii.

In the observations and arguments of those who
take the latter view of the subject, it appears to
me, however, that the immediate or exciting causes
have not been sufficiently distinguished from the
remote or predisposing causes. Although it is
generally true, that malaria fevers attack persons
after exposure to some of the ordinary causes of
disease, which have been mentioned, still it is
difficult to understand, why these fevers should be
an almost invariable consequence of the application of such causes, in some countries and situations, and rarely or never in others. There must
be some other cause to account for this striking
difference acting on the constitutions of the
inhabitants of such places generally. Whether
this predisposing cause consists in the effects of
the general physical qualities of the atmosphere
of certain climates or situations, (such as heat,
moisture, and the alternations of these,) which,
by gradually modifying the state of the body, predispose it to take on a particular form of disease
upon the application of a common exciting cause;
or whether the same state of body is the effect of a
specific poison emanating from the soil, and taken
into the system, appears difficult to decide. An
argument against the existence of a specific poison,
may be drawn from the circumstance of strangers
being less liable to be attacked by these fevers,
during the first year of their residence in a malaria

country, than afterwards.* But, on the other
hand, it may be said, that the powers of the
constitution are sufficient to enable it to resist the
operation of the poison, until they are weakened
by a residence of some time in the country.
However this may be, the circumstance goes to
show, that a certain period of residence in the
malaria site, is necessary, in general, to prepare
the body for its attack; and that there is no reason
for the fear, commonly entertained, of a sudden
attack of malaria, from simply passing quickly
through a malaria district. In some instances the
former view of the subject seems the most philosophical and rational; but, on the other hand,
there are such very striking examples of these
fevers appearing to be the immediate effect of
exhalations from the soil, as, in the present state
of our knowledge on the subject, we are unable to
dispute or controvert. Numerous examples of this
might be cited; but it may be sufficient to refer to
the sudden effects of the climate of Walcheren, on
our troops, in the ill-fated expedition to that place.

But if we are ignorant of the predisposing
causes, the exciting causes are in general sufficiently evident; and whoever passes the winter and

* This I found to be the case with the German, French, and
English artists, and others who reside a considerable time in
Rome. They were more frequently attacked with fever the
second or third years of their residence, than the first.

spring only in Italy, will, by avoiding these, have little to fear from malaria fever. This at Rome seldom appears before July, and ceases about October; a period during which few strangers reside there. The fevers of this kind which appear at other seasons are generally relapses, or complicated with other diseases. One of the most frequent exciting causes of this fever, is exposure to currents of cold air, or chills in damp places, immediately after the body has been heated by exercise, and is still perspiring. This is a more frequent source of other diseases also, among strangers in Italy, than is generally believed by those who are unacquainted with the nature of the climate. Long exposure to the direct influence of the sun, especially in the spring, may also be an exciting cause. This has certainly appeared to me to produce relapses. Another cause of this disease is improper diet. An idea prevails, that full living and a liberal allowance of wine, are necessary to preserve health in situations subject to malaria. This is an erroneous opinion; and I have known many persons suffer in Italy from acting on it. A deranged state of the digestive organs is generally the consequence of this regimen; and under such circumstances the individual is much more liable to disease of every kind. Irregularities in diet are among the most frequent exciting causes of this disease, among the peasantry about Rome, who are the principal sufferers from it. And I may add, that whether the stomach is disordered by excess in wine and animal food, or excess in vegetable food, it is of little consequence. A plain and moderate diet, as it is the most conducive to health generally, so it must, in the present case, best assist the constitution to resist the cause of this fever. If there is any one circumstance in the state of the constitution, which more than another enables it to resist disease, and to pass through disease safely when it does make its attack, it is, according to my observation, a healthy condition of the digestive organs. In every situation of life, and in every climate, this holds true.

In regulating the diet of persons living in a malaria country, regard should be had to the nature of the climate. The same stimulating regimen which might be borne, and even prove useful, in the damp, chilly atmosphere of Holland, will not be suited to the exciting climate of Italy. The peasantry in some parts of Italy are very sensible of this. While at *Fumicino*, near the mouth of the Tiber, one of the most unhealthy parts in the Roman States, Dr. Todd, on inquiring of the people what method of living they found most effectual in preventing this fever, was told that it consisted " in eating little, in drinking little wine, but that little of good quality, and in sleeping little during the day ; " and an eminent Roman physician informed me that he believed the most frequent exciting cause to be errors in the manner of living. Petronius recommends strangers who go to Rome in the summer to use a light cooling diet, "victu tenui ac refrigeranti utatur." Pucinotti attributes the severity of the Roman fevers in many cases to the use of bark, spirits, and other stimulants, which are by some used as prophylactics; and he relates the case of an old man, who had come from Romagna every second year to labour during the harvest in the Campagna of Rome, who never had the fever, and his beverage in the morning and through the day was cold water with a little lemon juice. This practice his father had adopted before him with the same success, but his two sons who would use spirits in the morning, both fell victims to the fever.* Sleeping with open windows, either during the day or night, more especially in places known to be subject to these fevers,

---

* Mi ricordo ancora d'un vecchio villano di Romagna solito a venire a Roma da deici anni, un anno sì e un anno nò, il quale non era mai incappato nelle febbri, e da me interrogato di che preservativo usasse, rispose : *invece dell'acquavite io ho sempre bevuto e la mattina e tra giorno grosse giarre di acqua col succo del limone. Mio padre faceva lo stesso, e veniva quivi medesimo, ed è morto veechio a casa sua nel suo letto. L'anno scorso io perdei due figliuoli in questa Roma. Questi matti, per quanto io li consigliassi, come quelli che erano stati militari, non vollero mai lasciare quella meledetta acquavita, che auzi vi ponevano dentro ora la polvere da schioppo, ora il pepe polverizzato. Essi mi morirono tutte due di febbre ; loro danno."* Della Flogosi; nelle Febbri Intermittenti Perniciose. Urbino, 1823. p. 17.

is very dangerous; and I have known repeated instances of fevers produced in this way. Towns are always safer than villages and the latter than country houses; and the central parts of a town are also safer than the suburbs.

Much has been said about the healthy and unhealthy quarters of Rome, and in this respect there certainly is a material difference in the summer; but in the season during which strangers reside there, this circumstance deserves much less consideration. More is to be feared from currents of cold air during the winter than from a confined humid atmosphere, which last is the evil to be avoided during the summer. This circumstance respecting the effects of different seasons, requires attention, inasmuch as a residence that may be very proper during the winter, may not be so during the summer.*

It may be stated as a general rule that houses in confined shaded situations, with damp courts or gardens or standing water close to them, are unhealthy in every climate and season; but especially in a country subject to intermitting fevers, and during summer and autumn. In our own country, nothing is more common than to see

* Verum urbis locorum, qui insalubritate culpantur, non eadem est toto anno, atque omni tempore conditio : æstivo namque, et autumnali tempore infames sunt; cæteris anni tempestatibus absque ulla insalubritatis suspicione incoluntur.—*Ratio Instituti Clinici Romani. Exposita A. I. de Matthaeis. Prefatio* p. xxv.

houses built in very unhealthy situations, a few hundred yards distant only from a good one. Again, houses in places otherwise unexceptionable, are often so closely overhung with trees as to be rendered far less healthy residences than they otherwise would be. Thick and lofty trees close to a house tend to maintain the air in a state of humidity by preventing its free circulation, and by obstructing the free admission of the sun's rays. Trees growing against the walls of houses, and shrubs in confined places near dwellings, are injurious also as favouring humidity; at a proper distance, on the other hand trees are favourable to health. On this principle it may be understood how the inhabitants of one house may suffer from rheumatism, headach, dyspepsia, nervous affections, and other consequences of living in a confined humid atmosphere, while their nearest neighbours, whose houses are more openly situated, may enjoy good health; and even how one side of a large building, fully exposed to the sun and to a free circulation of air, may be healthy, while the other side overlooking damp, shaded courts or gardens, is unhealthy.* The exemption of the central parts of a large town from these fevers is partly explained by the dryness of the atmos-

---

* Quibus etiam in locis (quod sane mirum) brevissimi intervalli discrimine, hic aliquantum salubris existimatur aer; illic contra noxius et damnabilis. Baglivi de Prax. Med., Lib. I., cap. xv.

phere which prevails there, and the comparative equality of temperature between night and day. Humid, confined situations, subject to great alternation of temperature between day and night, are the most dangerous. Of all the physical qualities of the air, humidity is the most injurious to human life; and, therefore, in selecting situations for building, particular regard should be had to the circumstances which are calculated to obviate humidity either in the soil or atmosphere. Dryness with a free circulation of air and a full exposure to the sun, are the material things to be attended to in choosing a residence. A person may, I believe, sleep with perfect safety in the centre of the Pontine marshes, by having his room kept well heated by a fire during the night.

It has been repeatedly asserted that the influence of the Malaria is increasing rapidly around Rome; and that, from this cause, at no very distant period the place will become uninhabitable. I could not discover any good grounds for this opinion during my residence there. Indeed, the malaria fevers were much less prevalent during the last five years, that I was at Rome, than they had been previously. This was attributed, and I believe justly, to the unusual dryness of the seasons. It is remarked that the number of these fevers depends upon the state of the weather during the summer. Dry summers give rise to few fevers, while rain in July and August soon fills the hospitals. In comparing the admissions into the S. Spirito, the largest hospital in Rome, (set apart entirely for males) during the last 25 years, I found that the number of fevers was not increasing.*

Persons attacked by this fever should be strictly confined to the house until the disease has been completely checked; and as soon as this is fairly effected, the sooner they change the air, the more likely will they be to avoid relapses, and to prevent a disposition to a return of the disease from being fixed on the constitution—a circumstance of great consequence to the future health of the individual. During the autumn or winter, such persons may go to Naples; if the spring is far advanced, Florence will be the better place.

The next circumstance connected with the diseases of Rome, which deserves notice, is the peculiar sensibility of the nervous system of its inhabitants. This is evinced, in a very particular manner, by the disposition to convulsive affections, and the singular sensitiveness of the Romans, especially the females, to perfumes. This peculiar susceptibility of the nervous system, appears to be of recent origin. We learn from ancient authors that the Roman matrons were fond of perfumes; and as this peculiarity is not mentioned by the Roman medical authors who have more recently written on the climate and diseases of

* See Table in the Appendix.

Rome, for instance Petronio, Baglivi, Marsilio Cagnato, and Lancisi, there can be little doubt that it did not exist in their time. "But in our times," says a modern Roman writer, "nervous affections, vulgarly termed *tirature* or convulsions, are extremely common, attacking females more particularly, but likewise delicate individuals of the other sex. So easily affected are such persons, that they cannot even bear the odour of the most pleasant flowers without suffering." In reference to the modern growth of this singular sensibility of nerves the same author adds : "This was certainly not the case with the ancient inhabitants, as they were accustomed to make use of very strong perfumes without inconvenience. Nay even in the beginning of the eighteenth century, much more in the age of Petronius, no such evils were dreaded, as no notice of the kind is found in authors; and we know, moreover, that physicians were then accustomed to introduce into the chambers of invalids of both sexes, with the view of purifying the air, the odours of flowers, plants and resins."* It is to be remarked that it is not disagreeable odours which produce such effects

---

* Nostra vero ætate nervosæ affectiones, vulgo *tirature*, seu convulsiones communissimæ sunt, fœminis præsertim, effæminatisque viris, quorum corpora a tam levibus causis commoveri solent, ut odorum licet gratissimorum vis ea facile perturbet ac male afficiat. Quod sane ignotum fuisse videtur veteribus incolis, qui maxime, atque innocue, odoratissimis

on the nervous system but the more delicate, and, to northern nations, agreeable odours of flowers, also vegetable and other perfumes. Hysteric headachs and numerous nervous affections are produced by such odours. As remarked by the author just quoted, this influence is chiefly felt by the females, though the males are not insensible to it. The Roman physicians, who agree in the recent growth of this morbidly sensitive state of the nervous system among the inhabitants of Rome, cannot fix upon any other circumstance, to which it can be fairly attributed, except the indolent manner of life of the Romans, which favours, especially in such a climate, the relaxation and sensibility of the system. Thus Dr. De Matthaeis, after remarking that powerful odours have at all times produced sensible effects on the system, observes, that "there is nothing wonderful in this, if we consider the daily increasing mobility of the nervous system, produced by the luxurious and inactive life of our Romans." * Such was most likely the principal source of this idiosyncrasy, and

---

substantiis utebantur. Sed neque Petronii ætate, neque inuente sæculo xviii. hujusmodi ab odoribus effectus pertimescebant Romani ; cum nulla de iis apud scriptores fiat mentio, et Medici ad cubiculorum aerem corrigendum florum, herbarum, resinarumque odoramenta utrique sexui passim, atque indiscriminatim commendabant."—*De Matthaeis op. citat.*

  * Nihil proinde est, quod miremur, si aucta in dies, a molli, nertique vita nervosi systematis in Romanis incolis mobilitate.

this no doubt still tends to maintain it; while the morbid sensibility of the nervous system once acquired is, doubtless, in some degree, transmitted from parent to child. But though much may depend on the effeminate and indolent manner of living at Rome, the climate, I believe, has some specific effect in inducing this state of the nervous system. The habits of the Romans differ little, I think, from those of the inhabitants of the other large towns in Italy, for instance, Naples, Florence, Genoa, &c. : and yet this morbidly sensitive state of the nervous system does not exist, by any means in the same degree, in these places. Even a temporary residence of some duration at Rome, produces a degree of the same morbid sensibility, and in cases where the Roman mode of living cannot be adduced as the cause. Something depends also, I believe, upon the moral education; though it must not be forgotten, that the sensibility of the nervous system in all warm climates is naturally more exalted than in the colder, and the influence of the passions far greater in producing and modifying bodily disease. This is particularly the case with the Romans; and, in tracing the causes of the chronic diseases of such of them as came within my observation, I was struck with the general reference of their origin to violent mental emotions.

Another disease, or rather class of diseases, of much more serious character, but also of modern

with enlarged and otherwise diseased abdominal viscera, the consequence of malaria fever.

Pure tubercular consumption is not of very frequent occurence at Rome, the greater number of chronic affections of the lungs being the effect of inflammation. These occur chiefly among the lower classes, who are badly clothed during the winter, and many of whom are predisposed to such affections, from having already suffered from repeated attacks of intermitting fever, which have left behind them obstructions of the abdominal viscera. In this way intermitting fevers, by inducing obstructions and consequent congestion of the abdominal viscera, may lead to tubercular cachexia and consumption. I found it impossible to ascertain the proportional mortality from diffierent diseases in Rome. The deaths from consumption were stated to me by an eminent physician of that city to be as few as one in fifty. But though I believe the proportion to be less at Rome than at any other large city in Italy, I am satisfied it is much greater than this gentleman believed.

Headachs are common at Rome, and among strangers I found them of very frequent occurrence. On the other hand, I met with several instances of habitual headachs in young persons disappearing during a residence there. In some cases the headachs appeared of the pure nervous character, but a large proportion of them originated in errors of diet, and were generally remedied by avoiding these. Persons subject to this complaint, especially if it is connected with irritation of the stomach, should be particularly careful of their diet at Rome, where, owing to the greater sensibility of the nervous system, slighter causes produce headach than in this country.

Rheumatism is not frequent. Chronic cutaneous diseases are less frequent than formerly. Acute cutaneous diseases, as measles and scarlatina, are generally speaking mild.

Among the diseases benefited by a residence at Rome, I may rank *Consumption*. In the early stages of this affection, I have generally found the climate favourable. I have frequently known patients who had left England labouring under symptoms that gave much and just alarm, (such as cough, expectoration, &c.,) which continued during the whole journey, and entirely disappeared after a short residence in Rome. The same persons have remained comparatively free from all bad symptoms during the whole season; and this when, from the ultimate result of the case, there could be little or no doubt of the existence of tubercles in the lungs at the time. In the advanced periods of consumption, I cannot say that the climate proved of any benefit, the disease generally proceeding in the usual course, and perhaps even more rapidly (especially during the spring months) than it would have done in

England. In some cases the disease was increased in a remarkable manner during the journey to Italy.

In *Bronchial affections* I found the climate of Rome very generally beneficial, especially in cases where there prevailed great irritability of the diseased parts, and of the system generally, with much sensibility to harsh cold winds. I have known many such patients who expressed themselves as feeling much better at Rome than at Nice, or any of the other places where they had resided. In chronic Bronchitis, indeed, more especially when the disease was of the dry irritable kind, or was complicated with irritation of the digestive organs, a residence at Rome produced the best effects; and in cases of this kind I am satisfied that it is the best climate on the continent. When, on the contrary, this disease is accompanied with copious expectoration, unaccompanied with much gastric irritation, the climate of Nice will generally prove more beneficial. Nothing was more common than to meet with bronchial diseases, which, after having been benefited by a short residence at Rome, were greatly aggravated by a visit to Naples, and again relieved by the return to Rome. *Chronic Rheumatism* I have also found much relieved by a residence here. I have not had many opportunities of comparing the influence of this city with Nice, but I had frequent occasion to remark

K

its superiority over Naples in this disease. Rheumatism in the chronic form, as I have observed
in another part of this work, is very frequently
consequent to, or connected with, a disordered
state of the digestive organs; and this must
be taken into account in selecting a climate for
persons labouring under this disease. On this
subject I must refer the reader to the article on
"Rheumatism." For persons disposed to apoplexy
or nervous diseases, Rome, of course, would not
be selected as a residence; nor is it proper for
persons disposed to hœmorrhagic diseases, or for
those who have suffered from intermittent fevers.

No city in the south of Europe frequented
by invalids, affords greater facilities for exercise
in the country than Rome. In the variety and
extent of its rides it indeed exceeds every other
large city I have visited on the continent. This
circumstance, together with the facility of egress
from the town, and the immediate vicinity of the
public walks to that part chiefly occupied by
strangers, render Rome a far less objectionable
abode for invalids than large cities generally are.
The Piazza di Spagna, and streets in that vicinity,
afford the best residences. The streets that run
in an easterly and westerly direction are better
than those running north and south, as they are
less exposed to currents of cold air during the
prevalence of northerly winds, and the houses
have a better exposure. Both the sitting and

bed-rooms of delicate invalids should, if possible, have a southern aspect. I had the temperature of several bed-rooms noted in the night and early in the morning, and I found a considerable difference between those exposed to the north and south. Nervous persons should live in the more elevated situations.

Besides care in the selection of apartments, there are other circumstances which require peculiar attention from the invalid residing at Rome. There is no place where so many temptations exist to allure him from the kind of life which he ought to lead. The cold churches, and still colder museums of the Vatican and the Capitol, the ancient baths, &c., are full of danger to the delicate invalid; and if his visits to these be long or frequently repeated, he had better have remained in his own country. When an invalid does venture into them, his visit should be short, and he should choose for it a mild warm day.

It is a grievous mistake to imagine that when once in such a place the evil is done, and that one may as well remain to see the thing fully. This is far from being the case. A short visit to such places is much less dangerous than a long one. The body is capable of maintaining its temperature, and of resisting the injurious effects of a cold damp atmosphere for a certain length of time with comparative impunity. But if the invalid remain till he gets chilled, and till the blood forsakes the surface and extremities, and is forced upon the internal organs, (among which the weakest will generally suffer the most,) he need not be surprised if an increase of his disease, whether of the lungs or of the digestive organs, be the consequence of such exposure. Once and again these visits may be made without any *evident* mischief; but sooner or later their evil effects will be manifest, as I have very often witnessed. The invalid, unwilling to admit the real cause in such cases, is too apt to impute to the climate that which, in truth, arises from his own imprudence and indiscretion, in exposing himself to causes which are not necessarily connected with the climate.

The period at which an invalid should arrive at Rome, when he has it in his power to fix this, is October; and if the chest be the part affected, and he is still morbidly sensible to the spring winds, the beginning of May will be sufficiently early for him to leave it. After this time he should move northwards, being guided by the weather as to the period of crossing the Alps; though this should scarcely be done before the middle or end of June. About the Lago Maggiore, or Lago di Como, the invalid may pass a week or two, if the weather is such as to prevent him from crossing the mountains. The Simplon is altogether the best passage from Italy to Switzerland at this season.

OF A SUMMER RESIDENCE.

For invalids who require to pass several winters on the continent, it becomes a matter of great importance to select a place where they may spend the intervening summers with the greatest advantage to their health. In doing this, two circumstances require consideration, namely the health and convenience of the individuals. For those invalids who have passed the winter in Italy, two plans present themselves—either to recross the Alps, or to select the most favourable situation in Italy. By the first, the invalid will escape the oppressive heat of an Italian summer ; by the latter, he will avoid the inconveniences of a long journey. In deciding between these, in individual cases, various circumstances will require to be taken into account, which can only be noticed here very generally.

Consumptive invalids in general will do well to quit Italy ; and I may observe that I comprehend in this class, not only those actually labouring under phthisis, but all such as are threatened by it, and have gone there with the view of preventing it. The summer heat of Italy will disagree with both in proportion to the advanced period of the disease in the former case, and to the deranged state of the general health in the latter. In both cases we generally find a weak and relaxed state of the constitution, accompanied, very often, with a morbid sensibility of the nervous system, in which great heat is always injurious.

Among this class of invalids some exceptions may however be found. To individuals of torpid constitutions, in whom there is little nervous sensibility, and little disposition to febrile excitement, with a defective state of the cutaneous secretions, and a rigid rather than a relaxed state of fibre, a summer in some of the more healthy and cooler situations in Italy may prove beneficial. As a general rule, however, the summer climate of Italy will disagree with all invalids labouring under general debility and relaxation of the system, or an irritable state of the mucous membranes, or who are disposed to diseases of the nervous system. And when symptomatic fever with morning perspiration has shown itself, this will afford a still stronger reason against a summer residence south of the Alps, whatever may be the disease.

Invalids should leave Italy before the great heat of summer, and must not return until this is over; that is, they should be out of Italy before the end of June, and ought not return to it before the end of September or beginning of October.

There may be cases in which the inconveniences attending this long journey, and those likely to arise from a summer in Italy, are so nearly alike, that it matters little which plan is adopted; and there are invalids, also, who may even pass a summer in Italy with advantage. Certain cases of chronic rheumatism, and of chronic affections of the mucous membranes, come under this class ; and also some nervous diseases—those, namely, which depend upon pure nervous debility, as some species of palsy, not connected with cerebral disease. But even these cases seldom bear a second summer in Italy. Indeed by far the greater number of invalids who have derived benefit from the Italian climate, during the winter, will do well to quit it on the approach of summer. This remark will apply more especially to those who labour under diseases of the nervous system, depending upon, or connected with, cerebral congestion ; indeed, very few of this class of invalids should venture to pass even the winter in a warm climate. Also, in cases of irritation of the mucous membranes of the lungs and digestive organs, and in congestions of the abdominal viscera, with a disposition to a deranged state of the liver, or to dysentery, the whole south of Europe will disagree during the summer.

The places principally resorted to by invalids, who pass the summer in Italy, are *Naples,* and its vicinity, *Sienna,* and the *Baths of Lucca.* These are the most eligible summer residences south of the Apennines ; nor do I know that any place superior to them, and possessing the necessary accommodations for invalids, is to be found in the more northern parts of Italy.

The preference to be given to any one of the places mentioned, will depend upon the particular circumstances of the case. Where sea-air is known to agree well, and where passive exercise on the water, or sea-bathing are advisable, Naples will of course deserve the preference—when no other objections occur to it; on the other hand, where there is much nervous sensibility, and when the effects of the *sirocco* are likely to prove injurious, Naples and its vicinity should be avoided; although the sirocco is not so severely felt at Naples during the summer as in the autumn and winter. But the baths of Lucca, and still more Sienna, will be better situations for such invalids.

VICINITY OF NAPLES.

The vicinity of Naples affords several beautiful situations, much preferable to the town itself, as summer residences. The *Vomero* and the *Capo di Monte* afford some good stations close to the city; and of the more distant ones, *Sorento* and *Castela-mare* are the best. Of these, Sorento appears to be the coolest; and this it owes chiefly to its peninsular form, being a long narrow strip of land, having the bay of Naples on one side, and the gulph of Salerno on the other. The only good communication between this place and Naples, from which it is distant sixteen miles, is by water; and this is a serious objection to Sorento as a residence for invalids requiring medical attendance.

Castelamare partakes more of the climate of the Apennines, and affords also their usual shelter of chesnut trees. From its western aspect, and the mountains which rise immediately behind it, this place enjoys a long morning shade; but its full exposure to the setting sun, renders the evenings often oppressively hot. The air is less dry also than at Sorento. There is a cold sulphureous mineral water at Castelamare, and many invalids from Naples visit this place during the summer, more on account of this water than its climate.

The island of Ischia is also resorted to as a summer residence, and it may deserve a preference by some invalids, on account of its mineral waters. These are very abundant; indeed almost all the water of the island is more or less thermal, and mineralized. No analysis of the waters of Ischia, nor any original work on their qualities, has been published, as far as I know, since the work of Andria.* The temperature of the hottest source in the island is 189° of Fahrenheit. That of the Gurgitello, where there is a bathing establishment, the most frequented in the island, is 144°.

---

* Trattato delle Acque Minerali di Nicola Andria. Napoli, 1783.

There are also natural vapour baths called *stufe,*
the vapour which supplies them rising through the
crevices of the soil.   This is conducted through a
number of apertures, so as to be directed against
particular parts of the body, in cases where partial
vapour baths are required.   The temperature of
the vapour in some of these stufe is as high as
120°.   Sand baths are also employed.   Professor
Daubeny, of Oxford, who visited Ischia while
collecting materials for his highly interesting and
ingenious work on Volcanoes, found the temperature of the sand 110°. two feet under the surface,
near the sea.*

---

* That gentleman did me the favour to analyze some of the
saline efflorescence which adhered to the walls, at the stufe
at Casamiciola.   He found 100 parts of this to consist of

Sulphate of Soda	51.0
Muriate of Soda	2.3
Carbonate of Lime	5.2
Silex and other earthy matters insoluble in water and in acids	3.6
	62.1
Water and loss	37.9
	100.0

This, though by no means given as an exact analysis, by
Professor Daubeny, may still be considered as indicating pretty
accurately the saline contents of these waters.   They also
contain some free carbonic acid.

The baths of Ischia are held in considerable estimation for their medical qualities, and are accordingly frequented by invalids during the summer, for the cure of ' various diseases. They are found very useful in chronic rheumatism, chronic affections of the periosteum, in the cachexia of pseudo-syphilis, in local paralytic affections, and in obstinate cutaneous diseases. The stufe are chiefly used in the latter affections. An hospital has long been established at one of the principal sources in the island, by a charitable institution at Naples; and many hundreds of sick poor of the capital are sent annually, in the months of July and August, to use the baths. Dr. Crawford, of Dublin, who resided a summer in Ischia, and paid particular attention to the cases of these poor patients, observed numerous examples of the beneficial effects of the warm and vapour baths, more especially in chronic rheumatism and in local paralysis. The waters are seldom used internally. Dr. Crawford considers Ischia one of the best summer residences in the neighbourhood of Naples. He found that the heat during the day was moderated by regular sea breezes, and that the nights were very pleasant.

There are also two mineral sources in the town of Naples, at San Lucia, which deserve notice here; one a light aërated *sulphureous* water, the other a light aërated *chalybeate*. The former is particularly esteemed by the Neapolitans, who use it abundantly, chiefly in the early part of the summer, the season in which it is most beneficial. It is very useful in Dyspepsia depending on an inflammatory state of the stomach. Cirillo, a celebrated Neapolitan physician, attributed the rarity of bilious diseases at Naples to the extensive use of this water. According to Signor Ricci, who analyzed this water a few years ago, it contains carbonic acid gas, sulphuretted hydrogen gas, sulphate, muriate, and subcarbonate of soda, carbonate of lime, and a trace of silex.* The solid ingredients are, however, in extremely small quantities.

The *chalybeate* water, which is also in considerable estimation, is rendered véry pleasant by the large quantity of free carbonic acid which it contains. The solid ingredients of this water, also, are in extremely small proportions. It is a light, pleasant, aërated chalybeate water, and as such will prove useful in the cases in which this remedy is indicated.

SIENNA.

Sienna affords a pretty good summer residence for persons who are not very liable to suffer from rapid changes of temperature, which often occur here, even during the summer, owing to the high

---

* Analisi Chemica dell' Acqua Ferrata e Sulphurea di Nipoli.

and exposed situation of the place. Sienna is considerably cooler than Naples, Rome, Pisa, or Nice. The annual mean temperature is 55°.60; being 6° less than Naples, and only about 5° more than London; but this arises from the coldness of its winter, which is only 1°.38 warmer than that of London. Its summer temperature is about the same as that of *Capo di Monte* at Naples, but 3° warmer than that of the Baths of Lucca. Its daily range of temperature is very great. It is a dry and healthy climate, and altogether a safe summer residence. For persons disposed to or labouring under pulmonary disease, however, Sienna is an unfavorable climate, at all seasons. For nervous relaxed people, it forms a better summer residence than either Naples or the Baths of Lucca. It is like the latter place exempt from mosquitoes. The saline mineral waters of *Chianciano*, the ancient *Clusium*, are at no great distance from Sienna.

BATHS OF LUCCA.

This agreeable little watering place, situated among the Apennines behind Lucca, is much frequented during the summer, partly on account of its mineral waters, and partly on account of the coolness of the situation : on this last account chiefly it is resorted to by strangers. The mean temperature of the summer here is only about

6° higher than the summer of London. In the middle of the day, however, the heat is often very great, but the evenings and nights are cool and pleasant, and there are no mosquitoes. June, July and August, constitute the proper season at this place. Earlier than June, and after August, the air is damp and unsuitable to delicate people. Their is some variety of situation; the *Bagni Caldi* are on the brow of a high hill; the *Bagni alla Villa* are partly on the declivity of a hill and partly on a plain; and the *Pont' a Seraglio* is in a narrow valley on the banks of the little river Lima. The Bagni Caldi afford the driest situation, and when protected from the sun, also the coolest. The vicinity of the Bagni alla Villa is warmer, but quieter and more retired. The accommodations, which have been greatly extended of late years at all these places, are pretty good.

The mineral waters of Lucca have a considerable reputation in Italy, and were formerly sent over the country in great quantities. There are various sources differing from each other chiefly in temperature; this varies from 86° to 128° (of Farenheit) or a little higher. At each of the sources there is a bathing establishment. The chemical contents consist of the carbonic, muriatic and sulphuric acids, in combination with magnesia, lime and alumen. These waters also contain a small proportion of iron, which, according to the opinion of Sir Humphry Davy, who examined the earthy matter deposited from them, is held in solution in the form of protoxide, by silex at a high temperature, but becomes decomposed on exposure to the air. The proportion of these ingredients is very small, and the water possesses no very active medical qualities. The Acqua della Villa is that chiefly used internally. Externally these waters are employed in the form of baths and of douche, in obstructions of the abdominal viscera, in rheumatism, in chronic paralysis and in painful spasmodic affections; and they are used very much in the form of injection in uterine diseases. The vapour arising naturally from the water, is also used in the form of bath. For all these means of applying the water, there are abundant accommodations in the way of baths, &c. The rides about Lucca on horseback are beautiful and varied; but there is only one or two drives for those who require carriage exercise.*

* For further information respecting this place, see Moscheni's work, *Trattato de' Bagni di Lucca*, 1792 ; and the more recent work of Dr. Franceschi, the present director of the Baths.—*Igèa de' Bagni, piu particolarmente di quelli di Lucca.* 1820.

SWITZERLAND.

Although I have not hesitated in advising invalids generally, and consumptive patients in particular, to quit Italy during the summer, I do not feel the same confidence in pointing out an unexceptionable summer residence, more especially for the latter, elsewhere. Switzerland in point of convenience certainly affords one very eligible, but much caution and prudence are required on the part of invalids labouring under pulmonary affections who remain there. The alternations of temperature in Switzerland are often very rapid and very considerable. The difference between the day and night is great, and there is often a sharpness in the air which proves irritating to sensitive invalids.

For those, however, who are merely threatened with consumption, the summer may be passed in Switzerland with safety, provided they use ordinary prudence. Such persons should be careful to avoid unnecessary exposure to the vicissitudes of the weather. They should also content themselves with such excursions only as do not cause them to be overfatigued, or heated at one moment, and exposed, while in a state of perspiration, perhaps, to a cold breeze the next; a thing which is constantly occurring during mountain excursions in Switzerland. They should neither take long walks nor climb steep mountains. In a word they should not for one moment lose sight of the object for which they are abroad, viz. the preservation of their health. They must not attempt to do every thing and see every thing like their more robust and healthy friends. Indeed they should avoid making excursions in company with those in perfect health, otherwise they may be led insensibly to do that which might prove very injurious to them, and this I have often found to be the case. In proportion to the weakness of their system and their liability to suffer from colds, should this class of invalids be cautious. One of the most rapid cases of consumption which I witnessed abroad, occurred in a delicate young gentleman who had exerted himself much in climbing the mountains of Switzerland during the preceding summer.

It will not I hope be supposed from any thing now stated, that I wish to throw obstacles in the way of young persons threatened with consumption taking exercise in the open air. This is so far from being my intention, that I think such persons can hardly be too much in the open air. All I wish to inculcate is, that they should be careful not to convert the best of all preventives into a source of evil. For this class of invalids, horse exercise is of all others the most favourable. I am convinced from experience that frequent and gentle motion through a mild atmosphere is one of the most soothing and invigorating measures which we possess, for allaying an irritated and congested state of the mucous membranes of the lungs, and improving the general health.

The borders of the lake of Geneva afford, I believe, the best situations for a summer residence in Switzerland; and the neighbourhood of Geneva is altogether the least exceptionable. Vevey is very hot during July and August. The higher situations about Lausanne are exposed to the north winds, especially the cutting Bise, which frequently blows in the evenings and nights after the hottest days of summer, producing a great and often sudden change of temperature. The low situations between Lausanne and the lake are close and hot.

For the consumptive invalid, whose symptoms already indicate a tuberculous state of the lungs, and to whom it is of the utmost importance to avoid congestion of these organs and irritation and inflammation of their mucous surfaces, no part of Switzerland affords, I believe, a very favourable climate: nor is it an easy matter to point out a proper situation. There are, in truth, so many circumstances to be taken into consideration in each individual case, that I find it most difficult to lay down rules applicable even to the generality of such invalids. For more particular directions, therefore, respecting the best climate for consumptive patients, I must refer to the article on " Consumption," in a subsequent part of this volume. I may remark here, that travelling in hot weather is highly exciting and injurious to all such persons; and almost any situation is better than a long journey during great heat. When the hot weather has commenced, which it does not generally do in Switzerland before the beginning of July, the consumptive invalid who finds himself in that country, will do well to remain there, selecting the best situation he can find about the western extremity of the lake of Geneva; not too near the water, nor too much exposed to the north. Such an invalid should live according to the rules of the strictest prudence wherever he resides. His great object should be to keep the whole system in a state of tranquillity, to maintain the functions of the digestive organs and of the skin in a healthy condition, and to avoid whatever could overexcite the circulation or irritate the lungs.

When a sea voyage can be obtained during the summer, it will, in many cases, be desirable, but not in the Mediterranean: the climate of the Atlantic is much superior in this respect.

In cases where the mucous membranes of the larynx, the trachea, or bronchia is the seat of irritation or chronic inflammation, and especially where this is complicated with a similar condition of the digestive organs, it will be desirable to combine with a favourable summer residence, the use of some mineral water known to exert a salutary influence over the diseased conditions of this class of membranes. In bronchial affections the waters of EMS, on the Rhine, of BONNES and of CAUTERETS, among the Pyrenees, and of MONT D'OR, among the mountains of Auvergne, have the highest character. For the more delicate and sensitive patients of this kind, the waters of Ems will be found the most suitable. For those who can bear a mountain air, Bonnes will afford more benefit, or Cauterets where the skin is partly in fault. Such invalids who have passed the winter at Nice, and mean to return there the succeeding season, will find among the Pyrenees a very convenient and agreeable retreat during the summer. In cases of long standing, in the more advanced periods of life, where a strong impression requires to be made on the skin, as in cases where it has been the seat of obstinate eruptions, and the disappearance of which coincided, in point of time, with the attack of bronchial disease, Mont D'or will, I believe, effect cures when the other waters will not.

The subjects of pulmonary affections, who have spent the summer in Switzerland, will do well to try the "*Cure de Raisins.*" Of the salutary effects of ripe grapes, taken in considerable quantity for some time, there can be no question. In irritation of the mucous membrane of the lungs and digestive organs, and in congestive states of the abdominal viscera, with a disposition to hæmorroids, ripe grapes taken, for some weeks, in the quantity of several pounds a day, with a light diet, and abstinence from wine and every thing exciting, will often prove very beneficial. On this subject the invalid will, of course, be directed by a physician on the spot.

In respect to invalids labouring under dyspepsia and hypochondriasis, some may spend the summer with the greatest advantage in travelling over Switzerland, while others will do better to take a course of the mineral waters of PLOMBIERES, of VICHI, of EMS, or of CARLSBAD (as the case may be) at their respective sources. But for further particulars on this subject, I beg to refer the reader to the article on " Disorders of the Digestive Organs."

I cannot close these few remarks on the choice of a summer residence without recalling the attention of the reader to the cautions I have already given on the subject of travelling. Unless a journey in hot weather is conducted with great circumspection, the irritation and excitement arising from it in susceptible systems (especially where any organ is in a state of chronic inflammation, however slight in degree) will do more mischief than any advantage that can be derived from a short residence in the best climate, or from the use of the most valuable mineral waters. It will be more advisable that such an invalid should remain quietly in a situation that is not the most suitable to him (but the inconveniences of which may, in a great measure, be obviated by prudence) than expose himself to the danger of having his disease increased by a journey in hot weather.

MADEIRA.

This Island has been long held in high estimation
for the mildness and equability of its climate, and
we shall find on comparing this with the climates
of the most favoured situations on the continent
of Europe, that its character is well founded.

The mean annual temperature of *Funchal*, the
capital of the island, is 64°, being only about 5°
warmer than the Italian and Provençal climates.
This very moderate mean temperature, relatively to
its low latitude, arises, however, from the summer
at Madeira being proportionally cool.   For, whilst
the *winter* is 20° warmer than at London, the
summer is only 7° warmer; and whilst the winter
is 12° degrees warmer than in Italy and Provence,
the summer is nearly 5° *cooler*.   The mean annual
range of temperature is only 14°, being less than
half the range of Rome, Pisa, Naples, and Nice.
The heat is also distributed through the year with
surprising equality, so that the mean difference of
the temperature of successive months is only 2°.41:
this at Rome is 4°.39, at Nice 4°.74, at Pisa 5°.75,
and at Naples 5°.08.

Whilst there is much equality in the distribution
of temperature through the year, there is no less
so in the progression of temperature for the day,
the mean range for the twenty-four hours being
10° by the *register* thermometer, while at Rome

it is 10°, at Naples 13°, at Nice 9° by the *common* thermometer, which gives only the extremes observed during the *day.*

The steadiness of temperature from day to day also exceeds that of all the other climates. In this respect, it is not half so variable as Rome, Nice, or Pisa, and is only about one third as variable as Naples. The degree of variableness from day to day at Madeira, is 1°.11; at Rome it is 2°.80; at Nice 2°.33 : and at London 4°.01.

The annual range of atmospheric pressure is also very small, being about the same as that of Rome and Naples.

Nearly the same quantity of rain falls annually at Madeira as at Rome and Florence, but at Madeira there are only 73 days on which any rain falls, while at Naples there are 97, at Rome 117, and at London 178. The rain at Madeira falls at particular seasons, chiefly in the autumn, leaving the atmosphere, in general, dry and clear during the remainder of the year.

From this comparative view of the climate of Madeira, it must be readily perceived, how great are the advantages which this island presents to certain invalids over the best climates on the continent of Europe. It is warmer during the winter and cooler during the summer; it has less difference between the temperature of day and night, between one season and another, and between successive days ; it is almost exempt from keen, cold winds, and enjoys a general steadiness of weather to which the best of these are strangers : the rains are circumscribed and generally fall at regular and stated periods. During the summer, that is, from June to September, the almost constant prevalence of north-easterly winds maintains the atmosphere in a temperate state. The sirocco, which occurs two or three times, at most, during the season, and then continues for a few days only, (seldom more than three,) sometimes raises the thermometer in the shade to 90°. With this exception, the summer temperature is remarkably uniform, the thermometer rarely rising above 80°. In consequence of the regular sea-breezes, the heat is not so oppressive as the summer-weather in England often is. Close, sultry days are little known in Madeira, and there is neither smoke nor dust to impair the purity of the atmosphere. Such, indeed, is the mildness of the summer at Madeira, that a physician, himself an invalid, who has resided for some time on the island on account of his health, doubts whether it is not more favourable to the pulmonary invalid than the winter.*

Autumn is the rainy season ; and towards the end of September or the beginning of October, the rains commence, accompanied with westerly or south-westerly winds. In November the weather

---

* See an excellent paper by Dr. Heineken, in the Medical Repository, vol. xxii. 1824.

clears up, and generally continues fine and mild till the end of December. Some snow usually falls about this time on the mountains and rain at Funchal, attended by north-west winds, and the weather continues more or less damp through January and February; but fog is never seen, and even during this, their *winter*, the thermometer at sun-rise rarely ever falls below 50°.

The *spring* at Madeira, as at all the other places, is the most trying season for the invalid, and will require even here a corresponding degree of caution on his part. In March winds are frequent, and April and May are showery.

The mild character of the climate appears to be accompanied with a corresponding degree of health in the inhabitants of Madeira. The peasantry, though as hard worked and badly fed as in any part of the world, are said to be as fine, healthy, and robust a race, as are to be seen in any country. This island is almost exempt from the diseases peculiar to warm climates, and little subject to many of those which are common in more northerly countries. Intermitting and remitting fevers are said never to occur, and continued fevers are rare; croup seems to be unknown; calculous disorders are very infrequent. The more prevalent diseases are cutaneous affections, and among these the elephantiasis. Apoplexy is also a very frequent disease. Bowel complaints are very common, and often fatal; and dysentery is said to be frequently epidemic. With respect to the prevalence of consumption among the natives of Madeira, there is a difference of opinion among those who have had the best opportunities of observing. " Though so highly beneficial in this disease, with the natives of other countries," says Dr. Gourlay, " it is not to be concealed that no malady is more prevalent here than Phthisis, with the natives of the island.* " Dr. Heineken's observation leads him to a contrary conclusion. " It has been asserted," says this gentleman, " that no malady is more prevalent than Phthisis with the natives of Madeira; but, as far as my own personal experience and the result of my inquiries go, I incline to a contrary conclusion." †

In my inquiries respecting the influence of the climate of Madeira on disease, I shall confine myself to consumption, which is, indeed, almost the only disease for the cure of which, Madeira has been resorted to. As I have never resided at this island, I must rely chiefly on the information and opinions, which I have derived from other sources. On this subject, however, I have obtained so much assistance from two English physicians, Drs. Heineken and Renton, who have long resided

* Observations on the Natural History, Climate, and Diseases of Madeira, by William Gourlay, M. D. 1811.

† Op. Citat.

there, (and whither one went on account of a pulmonary disease,) that the utmost reliance may be placed on the following observations. Both these physicians have published valuable papers on Madeira, chiefly with respect to the influence of the climate on consumptive patients. Their opinions regarding the propriety of sending such patients, in the advanced stage of the decease, to this island, are in perfect accordance with those I published on this subject, with reference to the Continent, nine years ago.* And the results of their experience, given below, confirm in the most conclusive manner, the principles which are inculcated in this work, respecting the proper period of sending consumptive invalids abroad. They show the necessity of adopting change of climate as a means of *preventing*, rather than of curing consumption. Dr. Renton, in a sensible paper published in the Edinburgh Medical and Surgical Journal,† makes some judicious remarks on the "inutility, not to say cruelty" of sending patients in the advanced stages of consumption, to Madeira. These he thinks called for by the increasing frequency of the practice, more especially as it is " evident that, generally speaking, the patient himself has nothing to do in the arrangement, and that it is principally in obedience to medical advice that he undertakes a voyage, productive of

---

* See "Notes on the Climate of France and Italy," &c. 1820.
† Vol. XXVII. 1827.

nothing but mischief and disappointment." "So uniform is the result of this practice," he adds, "that the annual importation of invalids from England is thought a fit subject for ridicule, among the boatmen, on landing these unfortunates on the island. *'La vai mais hum Inglez a Laranjeira;'* 'there goes another Englishman to the orange tree,' (the burying ground of the Protestants.)"

I give the following interesting and instructive table from Dr. Renton's paper. It is drawn up from the cases of which he had kept notes, during the preceding eight years.

Cases of Confirmed Phthisis . . 47.

Of these died within six months after their arrival at Madeira	32
Went home in summer, returned and died .	6
Left the Island, of whose death we have heard	6
Not since heard of, probably dead . . .	3
	—
Total	47

Cases of Incipient Phthisis . . 35.

Of these there left the Island much improved and of whom we have had good accounts .	26
Also improved but not since heard of . .	5
Have since died	4
	—
Total	35

" In the cases marked *Confirmed* Phthisis, there were copious purulent expectoration, diarrhæa, &c., and almost all of them terminated fatally.

" Some of those marked *Incipient* Phthisis were probably not fully entitled to an appellation so ominous. Their general character were young people who were said to have ' overgrown themselves,' and who had been subject in England to inflammatory attacks, having cough, &c. Others had suffered from neglected or mistreated inflammation, and in many there was a strong family predisposition to pulmonary disease. Most of them, I have little doubt, would now have been in their graves, but for the precautionary measure which was adopted. The other diseases (sent to Madeira during the above period) were asthma, scrofulous glandular enlargements and rheumatism, all of which were benefited by a residence here."

With respect to the consumptive cases which are likely to derive advantage from a residence at Madeira, Dr. Renton further remarks, " When it (consumption) has proceeded to any considerable extent, I should consider it the duty of a medical attendant not only not to advise the adoption of such a measure, but most earnestly to dissuade from it those, who, from hearsay evidence of the recovery of others in circumstances similar to their own, may feel disposed to fly to it as a last resource.

"That great and lasting benefit is to be derived even from a temporary residence in this climate, which is probably inferior to no other in cases where pulmonary disease is merely threatened, or where strong family predisposition to it exists; many living examples sufficiently prove. But even under such comparatively favourable circumstances, it ought to be strongly impressed on the mind of the invalid, that half measures are worse than useless, and that no advantage is to be derived from climate, however fine, unless it be seconded by the utmost caution and prudence on his part."

The result of Dr. Heineken's observations is quite in accordance with that of Dr. Renton. " Since the summer of 1821, about thirty-five invalids (I speak from memory and include those attended by other medical men) have either reached or sailed for this Island. Of this number two or three died on ship-board and three within a month of their landing; five or six just survived the winter, about an equal number lingered through the spring, and three or four entered upon and passed through a second winter. Of the whole number thirteen only, including myself, are now in existence.* Two of these were cases of asthma, and two of chronic disease of the trachea and larynx; if those be excepted, and these are con-sidered to be dead who cannot be alive three

* Dr. Heineken's paper was written in 1824.

months hence, the survivors of thirty-five or there-
abouts, in the short space of two years and a
half and who, so far from being cured, can only
make the best of a precarious existence, in a low
latitude, will be reduced to six."

This is a melancholy picture of the progress
of consumption under all the advantages of the
mildest climate; it shows in a striking point of
view the necessity of discrimination in sending
patients to Madeira, and ought to impress medical
men with a proper feeling of the heavy respon-
sibility which they take upon themselves in deciding
on a question of such importance. By far the
greater number of these patients should never
have left their own country; the advanced period
of their disease could leave no reasonable prospect
of benefit from such a measure, as is evident by
the result:—Of the thirty-five cases reported by
Dr. Heineken, several died before they reached
the island, three within a month of their landing,
and five or six in about six months. Of forty-seven
cases of the same class of invalids in Dr. Renton's
report, more than two thirds died within six
months of their arrival in the island.

The result of those cases sent to Madeira at
the proper period is very different. Of thirty-five
cases of incipient or threatened. phthisis, twenty-
six were much improved, and probably a large
proportion of these ultimately saved.

While therefore the result of sending *confirmed*

cases of consumption to Madeira shows the inutility of such a measure, to say the least of it, the effects of the climate on incipient cases, and those threatened with the disease from hereditary or acquired predisposition, are highly encouraging, and should lead medical men to recommend such a measure at the only time when it promises benefit.

When we take into consideration the high temperature of the winter, and the mildness of the summer, together with the remarkable equality of the temperature during the day and night, as well as throughout the year, we may safely conclude that the climate of Madeira is the finest in the northern hemisphere.

The salubrity of this favoured Island also—its exemption from all endemic diseases, and the general mildness of the ordinary complaints, from which no climate nor situation is exempt, contribute to render Madeira a very desirable residence for those invalids in whom benefit may be expected from a mild and equable climate.

There is no place on the continent of Europe with which I am acquainted, where the pulmonary invalid could reside with so much advantage during the whole year as in Madeira. On this subject I have already cited Dr. Heineken's opinion, which is of the greater weight as he himself resides in Madeira in consequence of a pulmonary complaint.

He has found that he rather retrograded during the winter, but always gained ground during the summer. " Could I enjoy for a few years," he observes, " a perpetual Madeira summer, I should confidently anticipate the most beneficial effects." So strong, indeed, is his opinion of the summer climate of Madeira, that he recommends pulmonary invalids, who can conveniently accomplish such a plan, to pass the winter in the West Indies, and the summer at Madeira.

The mildness of the summer of Madeira is a very fortunate circumstance for those invalids who require to pass several winters abroad, (which by far the greater number of consumptive patients should do,) and for whom it is very difficult to find a good situation during the summer on the continent, even after a long and often tiresome journey. When it becomes requisite for a whole family to remove to a mild climate, this is a consideration of much weight, more especially when the members of such a family are chiefly females. In Madeira, the invalid has only to change his winter quarters from Funchal to a more elevated situation in the neighbouring country. He is thus saved a voyage or journey, and if he is prudent, he will often find that he has gained more in health during the summer than he did in the winter. " As a permanent abode," says Dr. Heineken, in a written communication to me, " I believe Madeira surpasses every other, because it contains within

M

itself the means of equalizing the annual temperature more completely than any other spot with which we are acquainted. The *lowest* to which a thermometer exposed all night in a north aspect has ever fallen in Funchal during five years, is 50°, and the *highest* to which it will ever rise, at such a distance up the mountains as would in every respect suit an invalid, need never exceed 74°. The sirocco visits us so seldom, and its heat may so readily be avoided by closing the doors and windows, that it need not be taken into account. The mean annual diurnal range is from 8° to 10°, that is, from the extreme of heat to the lowest degree of cold; but an invalid may with a little common-place precaution, and without the aid of fires, live in a temperature never varying more than perhaps 6° throughout the twenty-four hours within doors. In a few words, I would say —there is no occasion for a person, throughout the winter in Funchal, to breathe, night nor day, within doors, an atmosphere below the temperature of 64°; or in the country, and at such a height as to insure dryness, above that of 74°; that he may during the summer take abundance of exercise by choosing his hours without ever exposing himself to oppressive heats; and that in the winter he need not be confined to the house the whole day either by wet or cold more perhaps than a score of times."

The foregoing evidence is quite sufficient, I

think, to show that where climate is likely to be useful in consumption, that of Madeira is preferable to any in the South of Europe; and it has this important advantage over all other places frequented by invalids, as I have already remarked, that they may remain there during the whole year without being subjected to the inconvenience of a long journey, or suffering from oppressive heat. When such consumptive patients only are sent abroad, therefore, as ought to be sent, a large proportion of them may pass the summer safely, and often even with advantage in Madeira. But I believe there are others of this class who would suffer from the summer heat even of Madeira, or at least would derive benefit from a cooler and more bracing air. They will generally be found among young growing persons, and more frequently females, of relaxed constitutions. To the more firm and rigid frame of the adult, in whom internal congestion is much more to be dreaded than relaxation, the summer at Madeira will often prove more beneficial than the winter.

But however adviseable it may be for an invalid who has passed the winter in Madeira to remain there during the summer, with a view of passing another winter,—a case will rarely occur in which it would be adviseable to send a consumptive patient from this country to pass the summer in that island. When such an invalid, however, has passed the winter in the West Indies, he probably could not select a better situation for his summer residence than this island.*

Although in my account of the climate of Madeira I have confined myself to its influence on consumption only, there can be no doubt of its being highly beneficial in several other diseases noticed in this work, more especially scrofula and bronchial affections.

The only part of Madeira where invalids reside during the winter, is Funchal and its immediate vicinity, which is the warmest part of the island. This advantage it owes to its being open only towards the south, while it is in a great measure screened from the north by the central mass of mountains which rise immediately behind it in the form of an amphitheatre. They who remain during the summer live in the country. The steepness of the whole island renders wheel carriages useless. Invalids must therefore ride, or be carried in palanquins or hammocks. There is abundance of horses, sure footed, and accustomed to the roads; the steepness of which are less objectionable to a class of invalids who ought to take their exercise chiefly on horseback at a moderate pace.

* It was my intention to have given some account of the climate of the West India Islands, as, I believe, they would afford a better winter climate, in many cases, than any of those which I have noticed; but as yet I have been unable to obtain sufficient information to satisfy myself on this subject.

The soil of Madeira is dry, consisting mostly of the *debris* of volcanic rocks. Provisions of every kind are good and abundant, and the water is pure and of excellent quality.*

Invalids intending to pass the winter in Madeira, should leave this country in the end of September, or the beginning of October. The beginning of June is sufficiently early to leave the island to return to England. The climate of this country is seldom sufficiently warm, or at least steadily so, for a consumptive patient who has passed the winter in a milder climate, before the middle or end of June—not until the summer solstice, I should say.

Opportunities of going from this country to Madeira are very frequent, as, independently of the regular traders, many West India vessels, and the monthly packets to the Brazils, touch at the island on the outward voyage. About ten days may be considered the average time of making the passage ; frequently it is less, and rarely exceeds fifteen days. The opportunities of re-

---

* The reader who is desirous of obtaining information on the natural history, &c. of Madeira, is referred to the writings of Von Buch, Bowdler and Gourlay, to the very interesting work of Professor Daubeny on " Extinct Volcanoes;" and to a small work lately published, " Rambles in Madeira and Portugal." Invalids intending to visit this island will find much useful information in the last named work, especially in the Appendix on the " Climate, &c. of Madeira," written by Dr. Heineken.

turning from Madeira are, however, by no means
so frequent; as comparatively few vessels touch
there on their voyage to England.   Yet I believe
that in this respect much inconvenience is not
experienced.

PART THE SECOND.

ON DISEASES.

INTRODUCTORY REMARKS.

BEFORE entering on the consideration of the various diseases, for the cure or relief of which a change of climate is recommended, I shall, in the present article, after taking a general view of the nature of such a change, and the extent of benefit which may reasonably be expected from it, endeavour to make the invalid acquainted with the various circumstances, which demand his particular attention, previously to setting out, during his journey, and after he is fixed in his new residence. This is a matter of the greatest consequence; and I am convinced that a want of due attention to it, is one of the principal reasons why much less benefit is really derived from climate than would otherwise be the case.

Too much is generally expected from the simple change of climate. From the moment the invalid has decided upon making such a change, his hopes are too often solely fixed upon it; while other circumstances, not less conducive or necessary to his recovery, are considered of secondary importance, and are sometimes totally neglected. Nor is the fault always confined to the patient; his medical adviser frequently falls into the same error: and it is not difficult to account for this. The cases hitherto sent abroad have been, for the most part, consumptive or chronic diseases, of long standing, in which the ordinary resources of our art have usually been exerted in vain, before such a measure is recommended. Therefore, when change of climate is determined upon, the physician, as well as the patient, is disposed to look upon it as the sole remedy. The former generally advises all medicines to be laid aside, except such as are requisite to keep the bowels regular; and with this counsel he consigns the patient to his fate; encouraging him to place his confidence in change of air, of scene, &c., and in these alone.

Such, generally speaking, has been the sum of the medical advice with which I have found most invalids sent abroad. And as I have witnessed, on a pretty extensive scale, the injury arising from this kind of over-confidence in the unaided effects of climate, and the consequent neglect of other things of no less importance, I particularly request the attention of invalids, (and I hope I may be allowed to add, of physicians,) to the following remarks.

In the first place, I would strongly advise every person who goes abroad for the recovery of his health, whatever may be his disease, or to whatever climate he may go, to consider the change as merely placing him in a situation the most favourable for the removal of his disease; and to bear constantly in mind that the beneficial influence of travelling, or of sailing, and of climate, requires to be aided by such a regimen and mode of living, and by such remedial measures, as would have been requisite in his case, had he remained in his own country. All the circumstances requiring attention from the invalid at home, require to be equally attended to when he is abroad. The necessity for such attention may differ somewhat in degree, but that is all. The same care as to regimen, exercise, &c. that would have been necessary at home will be equally so abroad. If in some things greater latitude may be permitted, others will demand even a more rigid attention. It is, in truth, only by a due regard to all these circumstances, that the powers of the constitution can be enabled to remove, or even materially alleviate, a disease of long standing, in the best possible climate.

It may appear strange to some of my readers that I should think it necessary to insist so strongly on the necessity of attending to things, which are so self-evident, and so consonant to common sense; but I have too often witnessed the injurious effects of a neglect of them, not to deem such remarks called for in this place. It was often, indeed, matter of surprize to me, during my residence abroad, to observe the manner in which invalids seemed to lose sight of the very object for which they left their own country. This appeared to me to arise chiefly from too much being expected from climate. Every invalid who goes abroad must make up his mind to submit to many sacrifices of his inclinations and pleasures, if he expects to improve his health by a residence on the continent.

The more common and more injurious deviations from the system of living, which an invalid should adopt, consist in errors in regimen; exposure to cold, over-fatigue, and excitement in what is called "sight-seeing;" frequenting crowded and overheated rooms, keeping late hours, &c. Many cases have fallen under my observation, in which climate promised the greatest advantage, but where its beneficial effects were counteracted by the injurious effects of these causes.

I shall now proceed to point out the circumstances which require to be more particularly attended to, in the general management of the invalid—previous to the commencement of his journey, while he is travelling, and during his residence in his new climate.

In order that the patient may derive advantage from his journey, or at least that his complaint may not (as often happens) be increased by it, some preparatory measures will generally be requisite before he sets out. Travelling is exciting to most people; and to those who have chronic inflammation of any organ, however latent or obscure, it very often proves injurious, particularly during hot and dry weather. Almost every one in health is sensible of the excitement arising from travelling. The appetite is generally increased on a journey, while the secretions and exertions are much diminished. The speedy consequence is a degree of excitement of the whole system, generally and not inaptly termed by travellers, "a heated state." What in health amounts only to a slight degree of excitement, easily removed by a few days' rest, and the employment of a few common cooling remedies, often proves of serious consequence to the invalid who labours under, or is even disposed to any inflammatory affection. The local disease, in whatever organ it may exist, seldom fails to be aggravated, under such circumstances; as is sufficiently indicated by a general febrile state, or the occurrence, or increase, of symptoms more immediately connected with it.

When, therefore, the patient's disease is of an inflammatory nature, or threatens to assume such a character, his condition should be well examined before he sets out. There should, if possible, be no vascular excitement at the beginning of a journey. If any local inflammation exists, measures should be taken to reduce it by proper regimen, by rest, by tepid bathing, &c.; and local or even general bleeding may be requisite in some cases. Simple congestion, or an overloaded state of the vascular system, general or local, will also require to be diminished. In short, before one step of the journey is taken, every thing like excitement or plethora should be removed, as far as the nature of the case admits.

Having his system in a proper state when he sets out, the invalid should endeavour to keep it so during the journey,—by adhering to a mild, light diet, taking care not to overload the stomach even with the mildest food, by abstaining from wine and spirits of every kind, and by maintaining the regular action of the bowels. The latter object is best effected, not by strong and irritating purgatives, but by laxatives, such as castor oil, electuary of senna, or of cassia, manna and mild lavemens. Purgatives of the more drastic kind, under which I comprehend nearly the whole class of *pills*, generally irritate the bowels, increase the disposition to constipation, and often induce hæmorrhoids; a frequent consequence of neglected or irritated bowels while travelling, To these means of maintaining the system in a cool state, I may add the use of tepid bathing, which should not be omitted where it can be conveniently procured, and when there are no objections to it from the peculiar nature of the patient's disease. When used at the proper temperature and with the necessary precautions, it is free from danger, and will generally prove very useful in obviating the exciting effects of travelling. The temperature may be from 94° to 97° of Farenheit's thermometer, according to the feelings of the patient. The forenoon, or, rather, just before dinner, is the best period for taking the bath, and from twenty minutes to half an hour the proper time for remaining in it. By adopting the general regimen mentioned, and by travelling only such distances daily as the invalid's strength can bear, resting for a day when he feels it necessary, he will not only avoid the injurious effects frequently produced by travelling, but will often find his condition improving as he proceeds on his journey, and will, probably, arrive at his winter residence in a much better state of health than when he left his own country. And this, I may observe, is a rare occurrence in the usual mode of conducting a long journey: for even when no positive increase of disease is the consequence, the traveller has frequently sufficient cause to regret his inattention to the precautions above mentioned; as there is often induced a degree of general excitement, and a deranged

state of the secretions, &c., the injurious effects
of which are felt by a delicate constitution during
a considerable part of the winter. The invalid
thus not only loses the benefit which he might
have gained by the journey, but that also, in
part, which he would have obtained from his
winter residence. If the invalid is wise, he will
keep these things in mind. It is the duty of his
medical adviser, as I have stated, to prepare him
for his journey, by reducing any excitement which
may exist in his system, and by removing any other
morbid affections with which the principal disease
may be complicated, and which often form in-
surmountable obstacles to recovery. And, having
his system thus prepared, the invalid should, on
his part, endeavour to maintain it in the same
state by a strict adherence to the prescribed regimen. If, during his journey, his pulse should
become frequent, his skin dry and hot, or if he
has thirst or a dry tongue in the morning, or if
his nights become restless, he may feel assured
all is not right. He is over-excited either by
too full a diet, by too rapid travelling, by exposure
to a hot sun, or by the bowels being overloaded.
In the generality of such cases, a few days' rest
and the use of some such cooling measures as
have already been pointed out, will restore the
system to its previous state; and the invalid may
then pursue his journey, taking care to avoid whatever he has reason to believe excited him before.

Arrived at his place of residence, some measures of the same kind will probably be necessary; as it will rarely happen, that one shall reach the end of a long journey, even under the best management, without some degree of excitement or derangement of the system. The invalid should, if possible, be spared the examination and selection of apartments, and particular care should be taken to have these thoroughly dry and ventilated before he enters them : this, I may remark in passing, is only to be done by the use of fires.

There are some other circumstances more immediately connected with the change of climate, which require to be noticed here. As the traveller advances to the south, the sensibility of the system is increased, and hence his mode of living requires to be regulated accordingly. Persons, for example, bear a diet in England which would prove too exciting to them in Italy : some articles of food, also, are more apt to disagree in the south ; of this kind are fish, milk, and even vegetables, all of which should be used in great moderation by persons in delicate health. As soon, therefore, as a person changes his climate, he ought to adapt his manner of living to that which he has begun to inhabit. Besides the diet, the clothing also requires very particular attention. The body ought to be fully as well covered in the south of Europe as in England. The feelings are very much altered in respect to cold, and houses being relatively colder in Italy, warmer clothing is necessary within doors than in this country. It is advisable, also, to keep the whole apartment of a moderate temperature, and to avoid approaching too near the fire. To seek also too exclusively the sun's rays is a habit injurious in the south of Europe, and more especially during the spring. From these causes arise headachs, catarrhs, inflammatory affections of the chest and even fevers.

This seems the proper place to say something of the best periods of travelling. With respect to the routes to the different parts of the continent, the ordinary *Guides* and books of *Directions* for travellers, particularly the comprehensive work of Mrs. Starke, contain such full information as to render it unnecessary that I should enter on that subject.

There are two seasons when the invalid who means to pass the winter in Italy may leave England,—very early in June and early in September. In setting out at the former period, he may pass the summer in Switzerland,—a plan which will suit the health and convenience of many. By leaving this country at the later period (viz. September) the intensity of the summer heat will be avoided, and, by conducting the the journey properly, the patient may enjoy a mild climate the whole way. But to insure this, nothing should be allowed to interfere with the steady prosecution of the journey, except such periods of, repose as the invalid may require. The best route will still be through Switzerland, and across the Simplon. The proper period for entering Italy is the end of September, or early in October.

For Nice and the south of France, it will not be necessary to leave England so soon, though the period of departure should not be much later. An invalid can scarcely have too much time for his journey; inasmuch as, if conducted with judgment, and made at the proper season it will be the more beneficial to his health the more time he occupies on the road, within reasonable limits. Water-travelling by passage-vessels on rivers, should be avoided, as exposing to great risk of cold from currents of air, &c. When the weather is chilly, the invalid should not commence his journey too early in the morning, nor until he has taken a light breakfast; and he should endeavour to arrive at his sleeping-quarters before evening.

One of the most exciting things to a sentitive invalid is exposure to a powerful sun, which should therefore be sedulously avoided, by resting during the middle of the day when the weather is oppressively hot.

When there is a disposition to coldness of the extremities, it is of essential consequence to the

N

well-being of the patient, to guard against this, by adopting the necessary measures to maintain the temperature of the feet, &c. When this cannot be effected by the ordinary coverings, the very useful and now common convenience of a vessel containing hot water, on which the feet can rest, should be adopted; and I may here add that this is an article, which an invalid should not go abroad without. When the surface and extremities are kept warm, a delicate person will often bear travelling in a very cool atmosphere, and even derive advantage from it. Persons with the slightest disposition to inflammation of the throat, trachea, or lungs, should avoid exposure to high wind or a strong sun, and, still more, alternations of these, which are very apt to occur in valleys, and in crossing mountains. Invalids should also avoid approaching too near a strong fire in the evenings after a journey.

The foregoing observations I consider to apply, more or less, to all invalids going abroad for the benefit of their health : for more minute instructions respecting the conduct of persons affected with particular diseases, and at different places, I must refer to the articles devoted to the consideration of such diseases and places, in the former and subsequent parts of this volume.

I shall now proceed to give some account of the diseases in which a change to a mild climate is adviseable.

DISORDERS OF THE DIGESTIVE ORGANS.

The great frequency, in this country, of what is commonly called "indigestion," "bilious," "stomach," or dyspeptic complaints, is well known; and the long train of suffering which they induce must be familiar to every medical practitioner. Nevertheless, there exists great discrepancy of opinion concerning the nature of the morbid conditions which give rise to these complaints; and hence the contradictory advice we daily find given to dyspeptic patients, and the unsuccessful practice of which we see them too generally the subjects. This commonly arises from practitioners overlooking the real nature of the disease, and directing their efforts rather to palliate symptoms than to remove the pathological condition on which these depend. It arises also, not unfrequently, from the attempt to find means of reconciling indulgences at table with the enjoyment of health,—a vain endeavour to bestow the reward of temperance on the epicurean.

In the remarks which I have to make on this subject, it will be my object to establish more accurate distinctions between the different kinds of dyspeptic affections: and although I cannot venture to flatter myself with the expectation that I shall fully succeed in my attempt, still I am not without hopes of being able to remove some of those discrepancies of opinion, and to correct some of those vague and indistinct notions, and partial views, which stand in the way of that method of cure which promises the only reasonable ground of success. Yet I am well assured that whatever may be done by any individual, in the actual state of our knowledge of the nature of these affections, there will still remain a large field for close and patient observation, before such a knowledge of them can be acquired as shall satisfy a conscientious practitioner. If we could succeed in establishing the true pathological nature of the diseases in question, we should have made the most important step towards the successful treatment of a class of disorders, certainly the most frequent, and, when considered in all their bearings, perhaps the most important of any to which mankind is liable. Unlike many others, these affections are productive of the worst consequences at a distance from their primary seat; and when neglected or improperly treated, they induce, sooner or later, a train of secondary disorders, which destroy the natural vigour both of the body and the mind; and too often reduce men of the most active, of the kindest, and most enterprising characters, to the most timid, irritable and helpless of human beings.

The morbid states of the digestive organs

exert an influence over the mental as well as the
bodily powers, which, although noticed by many
writers, is not yet fully appreciated by the profession, and is not even dreamed of by mankind
in general. I am convinced, however, after close
and careful observation, that the mind is more
generally influenced by the state of these organs
than by that of any other; and even that through
this medium are made the most frequent inroads
upon the integrity of the intellect.

The causes of dyspeptic complaints are numerous.
They may be arranged however under two classes;
those which exert their influence on the general
system; and those which act more immediately
on the stomach. Among the former may be
classed all causes which debilitate the body
and augment the nervous irritability—such as
mental anxiety, the depressing passions generally,
over-exertion of the mind, a sedentary life, a
residence in close, unhealthy situations, &c. But
the most frequent causes are those which act
directly on the organs of digestion. They are,
chiefly, errors in diet, and the abuse of stimulating
and purgative medicines, taken with the view of
correcting the effects of such errors. The former
class act more frequently as remote, the latter
more generally as exciting causes.

The morbid conditions induced by these agents
are of two different kinds :—(1,) an irritated state
of the mucous surface of the stomach of an

inflammatory character; and (2,) a highly increased degree of sensibility of the nerves of
the same part, accompanied mostly with a loss
of tone of the whole viscus. The latter affection
constitutes the proper, pure, or *Nervous Dyspepsia*; the former, for the sake of distinction,
may be called *Gastritic Dyspepsia*. Excesses in
diet are, according to my observation, the most
frequent cause of gastric dyspepsia ; whilst
intense and long continued mental exertion, a
sedentary life, a fluid relaxing diet, and constipated
bowels, give rise, most commonly, to the nervous
form of the disease. The manifest difference
in the pathological character of these two morbid
states shows, in a striking manner, the error of
applying the same mode of treatment to all cases
of disordered stomach.

The symptons characteristic of these two forms
of Dyspepsia, are often distinctly marked. In
the gastric or inflammatory species, the pulse
is very generally contracted, and often quickened,
especially after meals and towards night. In the
nervous species, the pulse is, in general, little
changed, though occasionally it is slower than
natural, and there is no disposition to fever.
Headach, which is so common and so distressing
a symptom of stomach disorders, is more constantly connected with nervous dyspepsia; and
its character differs also from that of the headach
which accompanies the pure gastritic form.

The headach arising from nervous dyspepsia, in its severer form, is generally preceded by a sense of coldness and creeping on the surface, particularly in the extremities, which sometimes amounts to shivering; nausea, or even vomiting, occasionally occurs at this stage : there is an insipid milky taste, with a clammy state of the tongue, and the pulse is slower than natural. In the commencement, there is rather a sensation of uneasiness than of actual pain ; but as the feeling of coldness diminishes, the true headach becomes developed. The pain then is intense and throbbing, and affects one side in general more than the other; the temples are most frequently the seat of the severest pain. The upper and back part of the head is also often affected; and the latter place is particularly apt to be so, when the headach is partly dependant on uterine irritation. During the continuance of the pain, there is great susceptibility of the nervous system.

In the headach which attends gastritic dyspepsia, the paroxysm is by no means so regular, nor so sudden in its attack. It is not usually preceded by coldness, but is often accompanied by a sense of burning in the hands and feet, and flushing of the face. The pain is of an acute character, and is also most frequently combined with a sense of distention ; the forehead and temples are its most frequent seat. It frequently terminates by vomiting. The period of attack is usually the evening, or during the progress of digestion; and whatever excites the stomach tends to bring it on, or increase it when present. The headach of nervous dyspepsia is more liable to come on in the morning than at any other time; often it begins on first awaking; and at all times it is more apt to make its attack when the stomach is empty, than during the process of digestion. Mental impressions, or causes acting through the medium of the nervous system, more frequently induce the nervous headach; though certain articles of food, which irritate rather than excite the stomach, are also a very frequent cause. Nausea and vomiting are more common in the gastritic; flatulence, vertigo, tinnitus aurium, deafness, dimness and other affections of vision, in the nervous dyspepsia.

In gastritic dyspepsia, the tongue is redder than natural, especially towards the extremity, and along the edges; in these parts it is also generally beset with small elevated points, of a still brighter colour It is also more or less furred. The fur increases towards the base, and the red papillæ, here of a large size, are often seen projecting through it. The tongue is often dry and parched in the morning and during the night. But these, and other appearances of the same part, are modified, in some measure, by the age and temperament of the patient; by the degree and duration of the irritation of the stomach, by the state of the bowels, and by the nature of the medicines which have been employed.

When the disordered state of the stomach has existed for a considerable period, the tongue often assumes a sodden appearance, and becomes as it were lobulated, with numerous fissures on its surface; in this case it is rather clean, or, if furred, it is in detached patches, the intervening spaces having a glossy aspect. This state of tongue I have remarked most frequently in persons who have lived fully, and been in the constant habit of using drastic purgatives.

In nervous dyspepsia, the tongue deviates less from the natural state, it is generally pale or covered with a thin white fur, but rarely dry. In some mixed cases, it has a swollen, œdematous appearance; and the impressions of the teeth are visible along its margins, especially in the morning. The gums, in gastritic dyspepsia, are often red, swollen, and spongy; and small apthous ulcers are apt to form on the tongue and lining of the mouth; and the fauces are habitually red, and often dry. In this species, also, there is more epigastric tenderness, and more disposition to thirst than in the nervous form. In the latter, the bowels are more obstinately costive, and the urine habitually pale, often very copious; and the extremities are usually cold. In the gastritic form, the urine is generally high coloured, and often turbid; the skin dry and parched, and frequently affected with eruptions; and the feet and hands, though occasionally cold, are at times unnaturally warm, particulary in the night. Nor are night perspirations during sleep at all uncommon. The face is apt to flush, generally or partially, especially after meals ; and the eyes, and still more the eyelids, are very subject to inflammation.

The sleep in both species is unsteady. In the gastritic form, when of some duration, the early part of the night is generally sleepless, whilst towards morning there is a heavy oppressive sleep, followed by a feeling of weariness on awaking, rather than the refreshment which succeeds to natural rest. In the nervous species, the sleep is better, but often and easily interrupted, and frequently unrefreshing.

The mind is affected in both cases. In the gastritic species it is more irritable ; in the nervous it is listless, frequently depressed and disposed to melancholy; but the most severe and obstinate cases of mental despondency, arising from a deranged state of the digestive organs, which I have witnessed, appeared more connected with the gastritic than the nervous form of the disease.

The effects of an irritated state of the digestive organs on the temper, is illustrated in a very striking manner in children, in whom they are seen uncomplicated with mental causes, to which they are in after life so generally, though often very erroneously attributed. Such a state of the digestive organs, when protracted, is a frequent cause of dulness in boys at school, by rendering them incapable of mental application. The head is often blamed on those occasions, when the stomach is more in fault. By too much and over-stimulating food at this early age, the mind, as well as the stomach, may be permanently injured. By the influence of long continued irritation of the digestive organs on the nervous system, at a later period of life, the disposition is often so thoroughly changed, the mind rendered so incapable of application, and the memory so much impaired, that the sufferer becomes unable to apply himself steadily to any thing, and is quite incapacitated for his usual avocations, and even unfitted for the ordinary intercourse of social life. Epilepsy, and insanity, generally of the melancholy character, are not unfrequent consequences of such a state, and in other cases it leads the unhappy victim to terminate his miseries by self-destruction.

Independantly of the particular symptoms which I have pointed out as belonging to each form of dyspepsia, there are circumstances in their general character which distinguish them. The symptoms which accompany gastritic dyspepsia, are more fixed and permanent; they may be present in a greater or less degree, according to circumstances, but they are never absent. In nervous dyspepsia, on the contrary, the symptoms vary in a remarkable manner. The patient feels, at times, almost intirely free from them, and the functions of the

digestive organs are performed with scarcely any
indication of derangement; or, all the symptoms
of the disease are often greatly augmented, the
patient being unable to assign any particular
cause either for their disappearance, in the one
case, or their increase in the other. Nervous
dyspepsia is also much more under the influence
of mental affections, of changes of the weather,
and other causes which particularly affect, the
nervous system; while the symptoms which characterize the gastritic form of the disease, are
more considerably and decidedly increased by
stimulants of every kind taken into the stomach.
The former is even sometimes temporarily relieved
by these latter means.

In mixed cases, these distinguishing characters
will be observed more or less as the one or other
form of dyspepsia prevails; for the gastritic and
nervous species of dyspepsia are easily con-
vertible into each other, and even frequently
exist together in the same subject. In this last
case, we have both the inflammatory excitement
and extreme morbid sensibility,—the one or other
state predominating at different times. Cases of
this kind are perhaps the most common, and they
are certainly the most difficult to treat. Yet
in all these mixed cases the leading characters
which show the prevailing nature of the affection,
are generally sufficiently distinct. Nervous dyspepsia, if long continued, generally terminates in

the gastritic species ; the latter, as far as I have observed, rarely changes permanently into the former.

Complicated with, and generally consequent to the morbid conditions of the mucous surface of the stomach, there is very generally a congested and embarrassed state of the abdominal circulation, and a diminished, and generally depraved secretion from the mucous membrane of the bowels, from the liver, and other secreting organs connected with digestion. Such complications often tend to render the case obscure, and the treatment a matter of great nicety and delicacy.

In the uncomplicated cases of dyspepsia, and especially in their early stages, the cure is not in general difficult, provided the exciting causes can be withdrawn, and the disorder is treated upon rational principles. It is very different, however, when the disease has been of long standing; its removal then requires great resolution and perseverance on the part of the patient, and much judgment and patience on the part of the physician. In protracted cases, the disorder is seldom confined to the stomach : it is gradually propagated to the mucous membranes of other parts ; to the intestines, to the throat, to the trachea, the bronchia, kidneys, bladder, urethra, or uterus ; and often, from the mucous membranes of these organs the irritation is transferred to the

glands more immediately connected with them,—
to the liver, testes, mammæ, &c.

Of these secondary affections, that of the liver
is one of the most frequent. But although a
congested state of the vessels, and a deranged
condition of the secreting functions of this viscus,
are very constant attendants on dyspepsia of some
duration, the liver is much more rarely diseased
than is generally believed. The common expressions of the liver being " affected," " touched,"
&c., so generally employed in cases of dyspepsia,
are to be regarded as words without any definite
meaning being attached to them, even by those
who use them ; and are too often, I fear, employed
to conceal our ignorance of the nature of the
disease. On this account, these indefinite expressions deserve condemnation ; but I notice
them here chiefly to deprecate the mischievous
practice to which they too often lead. I allude
to the indiscriminate use of mercury, in the form
of calomel or blue pill, &c., and of irritating purgatives. This is a mode of treatment which,
notwithstanding its very general employment, I
think I may venture to say never yet cured a
single case of dyspepsia ; and I am satisfied that
in this disease, it has been, and continues to
be, productive of incalculable mischief; more
especially in females, in delicate constitutions
generally, and in young children. It is true,

such practice frequently affords a temporary relief, more especially when it produces a copious secretion from the liver; but when mercury is long continued, even in small doses, or frequently repeated in larger doses, it very often fixes the disease on the mucous surface of the digestive organs, and through them excites an irritation in the whole nervous system that is never entirely removed. This is more especially the case in the nervous forms of dyspepsia, and in persons naturally of a very sensitive nervous system.

During my residence on the continent, I met with many victims to the abuse of mercury in its various forms, among the invalids who annually came to Italy—sent abroad, in too many instances, after the constitution was reduced to such a shattered state that no climate or mode of life could materially improve. Indeed, I may safely affirm, that among the numerous cases of decayed constitutions, which I met with among dyspeptic invalids, the larger proportion had suffered more from calomel and drastic purgatives, than they would have done, I believe, from the disease if left to itself. Calomel is a valuable remedy when used with judgment and discretion, but it is one of the most destructive agents of. the materia medica in the hands of persons ignorant of its real operation. When the nature of dyspeptic complaints is better understood, mercury will not be employed, more espe-

cially in the nervous form of the disease, once in
a hundred times so frequently as it is at present.

But to return from this digression. We often
find that the diseased state of the stomach, in
place of being propagated to the internal surfaces of other organs, is translated to other
systems. It is thus that we find it producing
various affections of the skin and of the nervous
system. Among the last may be mentioned
different convulsive disorders, tic douloureux,
paralysis, amaurosis, deafness, loss of smell, loss
of voice, asthma, palpitation, &c.; and, in the
more exquisite degrees, I believe, in some cases,
it ultimately leads to diseased structure of the
brain, and, as a consequence, to permanent
epilepsy, to palsy, to apoplexy, or to confirmed
mania. In other instances, it induces functional, and even organic disease of the heart.
Gout is well known to originate in an irritated
condition of the digestive organs; and rheumatism
also frequently depends upon this state. Many
of these symptomatic disorders simulate idiopathic
affections of the same kind, so perfectly as to
be often erroneously treated as such.

The nature of the secondary affection depends
often, I believe, upon peculiarities of constitution;
but frequently, also, upon accidental causes, exciting or disposing to these diseases during the
existence of dyspepsia. The new disease being
ingrafted on the old, becomes as it were dependant

on it, and the former cannot be cured till the
latter is removed.

It is a curious and interesting subject of inquiry
—what secondary affections originate in the gastritic, and what in the nervous form of dyspepsia;
but the consideration of this would carry me
beyond the object of the present remarks. It is
certainly true, that, as the secondary disease
becomes established, the primary affection is
mitigated, at least for a time. Indeed, so remarkably is this the case, that the primary disease is
often overlooked, both by the patient and his
medical attendant, amid the more prominent
symptoms of the secondary affection. This I
found to be very frequently the case in patients
sent abroad labouring under chronic bronchial
and tracheal irritation, symptomatic of gastric
disease.

In the more complicated and protracted cases
of dyspeptic disease, we have to combat a state
of constitution in which the remedial indications
often seem almost to contradict each other. We
have an irritated and irritable state of the
mucous surfaces; a congested state of the internal
blood vessels, and particularly of those of the
abdomen; a diminished circulation through the
surface and extremities; and, very generally, a
morbidly sensitive state of the whole nervous
system, with depression of spirits, or great irritability of mind, or both. We have constitutional

irritation which requires soothing; an irregular distribution of the circulating fluids, and of the nervous influence which requires to be regulated; diminished, disordered, or suppressed secretions which require to be increased, corrected, or restored; and all this often with such a broken state of constitution, mental as well as physical, as affords little help to our therapeutical means in promoting the process of restoration. Cases of this kind, in the more exquisite forms, fell under my observation annually, among the invalids sent to Italy from this country.

Among the remedial measures for these various morbid conditions, whether in their primary or secondary forms, there is none which affords a fairer prospect of relief than a change of climate. It is true, this remedy is not at the command of many sufferers from these complaints, but I believe it is a matter of much easier attainment than is generally imagined. At all events, it is attainable by that class in whom the disease now under consideration most frequently occurs. Even when the patient cannot avail himself of so complete a change of climate as we have been contemplating, he may still derive much benefit from a residence in some of the most favourable situations which have been pointed out in our own island.

In recommending such a change, however, to the dyspeptic invalid, the peculiar disorder of the

stomach must be attended to. The two opposite
states of the disease, noticed above, require different climates. The patient with well marked
gastritic dyspepsia should not, for example, go to
Nice nor the south-east of France. In cases of this
kind, Pau, or some other part of the south-west of
France, or even Devonshire, would be preferable.
Rome and Pisa are the best places in Italy for
such a patient. On the other hand, when nervous
dyspepsia predominates, and there exist languor
and sluggishness of the system, as well as of the
digestive organs, with more settled lowness of
spirits and hypochondriasis,—a state of mind rather
of a sombre desponding cast, than of an angry,
complaining character—and when the pulse is slow
and the feelings blunter, Nice is to be preferred to
all the other places mentioned; and in the same
cases, Naples will generally agree better than Pisa
or Rome.

In the more complicated and protracted cases,
still more discrimination is required in selecting the
best climate and residence; as we must take into
consideration not merely the character of the
primary disorder, but the state of mind with which
it is accompanied, and the nature of the secondary
affection which may already exist, or to which the
patient may be predisposed. It is surprizing what
slight changes of situation affect this morbidly
sensitive class of patients.

To insure the full advantages to be derived from

the best chosen climate, in such cases, urgent symptoms should be removed or alleviated before the patient commences his journey; and he should, moreover, have the nature of his disorder, and the principles upon which he should regulate himself, on his journey and during his residence abroad, fully explained to him. The want of due attention to these things, is one of the chief reasons why dyspeptic invalids often derive little advantage from their summer tour, or even from a more protracted residence abroad. In order to secure success to our prescription of a change of air or climate, it is necessary, also, that the patient should understand the conditions on which the promise of relief is made, and how they are to be best and most perfectly fulfilled. Above all, it should be im-presssed on his mind, that he is not to expect too much from climate; that he must sedulously avoid the causes which brought on the disease, and adhere with steadiness to such a general regimen as is necessary for its removal. Aided by this moral and medical discipline, a winter spent in a favourable climate cannot fail to prove highly beneficial to the dyspeptic invalid; and a well applied course of mineral waters, the following summer, will, in many cases, be of the greatest service in restoring the impeded functions of the abdominal viscera and of the skin. After this, the patient may return with a degree of bodily health and of mental energy to which he has long been a stranger; and may continue to reap the fruits of his perseverance and self-denial, so long as he shall avoid the exciting causes of the disease.

The extent to which change of air or climate requires to be carried for the removal of stomach complaints, will depend on the circumstances of the case. In many instances, a few months—even a few weeks judiciously employed, will do much for the restoration of the health; in others, a much longer period will be required. In treating, therefore, of the influence of change of climate and change of air in dyspeptic disorders, it will be both convenient and useful to divide them into two classes,—the more recent and simple, and the more protracted and complicated cases.

1. I shall first make a few remarks on the former class of patients, in which is comprehended that numerous body of our citizens, and the inhabitants of large towns generally, whose general health, and digestive organs in particular, have suffered by a sedentary life, close application to business, errors in regimen, &c., during the winter, and who require change of air during the summer, in order to enable them to meet the labours of the succeeding season.

The plans generally adopted with this view, are a residence during the summer months at some of our watering places, or a tour through the mountainous parts of our own island, or on the continent,—and more particularly in Switzerland. The preference which one or the other of these means deserves, will depend upon the nature of the case, the convenience of the patient, and various other circumstances, which can only be appreciated by the patient himself, and his physician.

We shall suppose that a tour is the measure adopted. Having had the more urgent symptoms of his complaint removed or alleviated, before he sets out, by proper regimen,* the next object of importance with the dyspeptic traveller is diet. This must be regulated according to the state of the digestive organs, regard being had to the exciting effects of travelling (pointed out in a former part of this work,) which render more especial attention to the diet necessary during a journey. If much gastric irritation exists, and, more especially, if this is accompanied with any disposition to fever, the diet should be very mild and very moderate in quantity. A small proportion of animal food, once a day, is all that should be allowed in such cases; and this should be taken in the middle of the day, or, at least, not at night. Tea or arrow root, sago, or gruel, form the best evening meal. Eggs and fish are improper food in such cases, and should therefore rarely be used. The best general drink is toast-water; and

---

* See Introductory Remarks to Part Second.

wine and all kinds of fermented liquors and spirits should be entirely avoided by the greater number of dyspeptic patients, while travelling. In those cases in which there is less of irritation and excitement, a fuller diet may be allowed, but in all cases it should be moderate in quantity, and of a mild unirritating quality.

I am aware that in travelling on the continent, it is not always a very easy matter to obtain that kind of food which is suited to irritable or delicate stomachs; but by a little management on the part of the traveller, this difficulty may be obviated in a great degree. By taking a little cold meat and good bread with him whenever he meets with them, he renders himself independent of the fare he may obtain at the smaller inns. Some rice or vermicelli soup may, in general, be procured, a dish which does not always deserve the contempt in which it is generally held by English travellers. The soups of the continent, if not so strong, are generally more wholesome and agree much better with weak and irritable stomachs than the rich compound soups of this country; and the opinions commonly entertained in England respecting soup in dyspeptic affections, are not applicable to all soups. Ripe fruit may be occasionally indulged in, but with great moderation, as it will seldom be found to agree in either form of stomach complaint; it is safer when dressed.

If the dyspeptic invalid will only observe the

effects which the different articles of food produce, and be true to himself and candid in his observations, he will soon discover that the more moderately he lives the better he will feel. When he has passed a restless night, or has a dry or loaded tongue, or bitter taste in the morning, he may be assured, that the regimen of the preceding day was not suited to him,—that he has erred either in the quantity or quality of his food, and should regulate himself accordingly for the future.

The next circumstance requiring the particular attention of the dyspeptic traveller, is the state of the bowels. Constipation is an evil from which travellers generally, and more especially dyspeptics suffer; and it is of great consequence that this state should be obviated. The mild diet which has been recommended will be a means of favouring the action of the bowels, and of moderating the injurious effects of their inaction when this occurs. For the removal of constipation, the milder laxatives are much safer and more effectual than the irritating drastic purgatives. The latter, even when given in the smallest doses, irritate the stomach and bowels, and, in this way, are often productive of more mischief than the state they are intended to obviate, which state their frequent repetition tends, moreover, to confirm. Castor oil, or confection of senna, or manna, taken in such doses only as is found sufficient to obviate constipation, are the best medicines. They may be taken at bed time, so as to act the following morning. But what often answers much better than any aperient medicine is the use of mild lavemens. To persons who have very sensitive bowels, and who suffer from constipation, lavemens prove an invaluable remedy on a journey, and, more especially to females; and no one should travel without being provided with the means of relieving the bowels in this way. The relief obtained by the judicious use of this remedy, will not only add greatly to the comfort of the patient, but favour the return of the bowels to a more healthy and regular performance of their functions; while it will obviate the necessity of having frequent recourse to purgative medicines, a fruitful source of mischief, as I have already remarked, to dyspeptic invalids. The lavemens should consist of water, barley water, oatmeal water, or thin gruel, tepid. Where these simple lavemens fail, a little honey, with or without the addition of some olive oil, or a little salt, or electuary of senna dissolved in the lavement, will occasionally answer; when these ingredients are added, a smaller quantity of fluid should be used. Perfectly cold water proves very beneficial in some cases, but soap and all stimulating ingredients given in this way generally disagree.

Tepid bathing is a remedy that should never be neglected by the dyspeptic invalid while travelling. It clears the surface, promotes cutaneous secretion, and tends to equalize the circulation, while it cools and soothes the whole system. The manner of taking the bath has been already noticed.*

If the dyspeptic invalid will attend to these simple directions, I will venture to promise him much greater and more lasting benefit from his tour than he would otherwise have derived. Let the healthy and robust boast of the thousands of miles they have travelled in a few months, and of the excellent wines and dinners they have enjoyed, but let the delicate and valetudinarian traveller keep in mind that he has a more important object in view, that health is only to be regained by such a rate of travelling as is commensurate with his strength, and by strict adherence to such a regimen as comports with the deranged state of his system.

These observations, which have been more especially addressed to travellers on the continent, are equally applicable to those who confine their excursions to our own island, or who pass some time at the sea-side or inland watering places during the summer. Those who visit the sea-coast will find the tepid sea-bath a valuable remedy. With a few dyspeptics cold sea-bathing may agree, but will not suit in many cases. The cold shower bath is better, and will be found more generally beneficial. But the warm or tepid bath will prove

* See Introductory Remarks to Part Second, p. 172.

beneficial in almost every case; and the vapour bath, also, will prove very serviceable in certain cases, more especially where the skin has been long in a dry state. But in all such cases, it should be impressed on the patient's mind, that it is in vain to expect that any kind of bath, or any remedy, will restore the skin to a healthy state, while the irritation of the digestive organs is kept up by improper diet. The dry state of the skin is consequent upon an irritated state of the internal surfaces, and until this is removed the natural state of the skin cannot be restored. Without attention to this, the vapour bath will be of little use and may prove injurious.

The great and common errors in these cases are, as I have already said, the condition in which invalids are sent to those places, and the manner in which they live while there. Much greater and more permanent benefit would be derived from a change of air, were its effects aided by such remedial measures and such a regimen as the nature of the case required. As matters are generally managed at present, the invalid has frequently not returned many weeks, when he finds himself in the same state as when he left his home. The reason of this is sufficiently evident. Previously to the tour, little or nothing is done for the mitigation of the disorder of the digestive organs, and no system of regimen is adopted by which the beneficial effects of change of air, &c.

might be favoured and rendered more permanent. All is trusted to air, relaxation from business and amusements ; and when the influence of these is withdrawn, the dyspeptic and nervous invalids lapse rapidly into their former state.

2. I come now to make a few remarks on the more protracted and complicated cases of dyspepsia, in reference to change of climate. Persons whose digestive organs have been long deranged, and upon whose constitutions great inroads have been made, will require a longer period of residence in a mild climate ; as, without this, they cannot expect much or lasting benefit. The impressions produced by causes operating for a series of years on the stomach, and through it on other important organs and on the system generally, are not to be obliterated by a residence of a few months in the best climate, even when assisted by the most judicious regimen, and the most exemplary conduct on the part of the patient.

Generally speaking, such invalids will derive benefit by changing our own damp, chilly climate for a drier and milder one, during the winter. But it is not a matter of indifference in what place they fix their abode ; and, indeed, it was the consideration of this circumstance chiefly, which induced me to go somewhat into detail, in endeavouring to describe the distinguishing characters of the different affections of the stomach.

I have pointed out two leading forms of disorders of the digestive organs:—one, in which there is an inflammatory state of their mucous surfaces; the other, in which a morbidly sensitive state of these organs is the principal feature, and which is also, for the most 'part, accompanied with a languid and torpid condition of the digestive function, and a congested state of the abdominal venous system. This is an important distinction, and must never be lost sight of by those who really desire to acquire a correct knowledge of dyspeptic complaints, and to be able to treat them on rational principles.

It is true, as I formerly observed, these two morbid states pass into each other in every variety of shade, from the pure gastritic dyspepsia on the one hand, to the pure nervous dyspepsia on the other; and the successful management of each case, will much depend upon the degree of discrimination exercised in referring it to its proper place in the scale. And this applies as much to change of climate, as to any other remedy. In the first class, in which there is a degree of gastric irritation, the climate of Rome will prove one of the best in Italy, and that of Nice one of the worst. On the other hand, where the nervous system is chiefly affected,—where there is a greatly embarrassed abdominal circulation, with a disposition to mental despondency, Rome will not, in general, agree. The climate of Nice in this case will be more suitable. Even the selection of a residence in the same place is not a matter of indifference to very sensitive invalids. One will feel himself better in an elevated situation, another in a lower and more sheltered one. The high and low and more confined situations of Rome and of Naples, afforded me many opportunities of observing the different effects of locality on such persons, and satisfied me of the necessity of attending to this circumstance, in selecting a residence for them. But dyspeptic patients, who pass the winter in Italy, need not in general be confined to one place; they may visit during the season the principal cities in the south of Italy; and if this is done with prudence, the successive changes may prove beneficial to their health; although the climate most suited to the particular character of their complaint should be selected as their principal residence. Generally speaking, Rome will be the best residence in Italy in gastric dyspepsia, especially during the spring.

To all these patients the spring proves the period of the greatest excitement; and they who are disposed to the more acute kind of stomach affections, must be more particularly on their guard against whatever can excite the digestive organs at this season. The same degree of stimulus that is tolerated in the winter, will prove injurious to them in the spring.

In mucous irritations, whether of the digestive

or pulmonary organs, I had every year occasion to remark the increase of excitement that occurred during the spring months. At this season there are great and often rapid alternations of temperature, which are extremely exciting to sensitive invalids. A powerful sun, frequently accompanied with sharp winds during the day, alternates with cold nights. This may be said to be the character of the spring generally; but in the south of Europe it is particularly so, and this circumstance renders the climate injurious in the more acute degrees of gastritic dyspepsia.

But it is not, as I formerly observed, for the more acute forms of dyspepsia, that I am now recommending a change of climate;—but for the chronic affections of long standing, in which the more acute and subacute stages have passed over, and, with them, the highly excitable state of the digestive organs. For these, and for the essentially chronic cases of nervous dyspepsia, particularly when accompanied with hypochondriasis, a residence for some time in the south of Europe will be of the greatest service, under the limitations, however, pointed out with respect to season, residence, regimen, &c. For the hypochondriac more especially, whose mind is likely to feel an interest in the variety of scenes, and the objects of art which present themselves so abundantly in Italy, I know no measure more likely to prove beneficial. I class the hypochondriac with the

dyspeptic patients; because, without venturing to
affirm that the former is always a consequence
of the latter, I think I can safely state that it is
very rarely met with unaccompanied with more
or less of dyspepsia; and, in a large proportion
of cases, it acknowledges the same origin, and
is cured by the same means.

Though such patients, therefore, should not
be encouraged to dwell on their complaints and
attend to every trifling sensation, I consider it
essentially wrong to send them abroad with the
assurance that their complaints are merely imaginary,—that change of air, of scene and amusement, will dispel their gloomy thoughts and
restore their feelings of health, and that nothing
else is required for their cure. This may be
very agreeable information to the friends of a
desponding dyspeptic. It is also a very easy
way for the physician to get out of an obscure
case; but it is seldom the way to cure the patient.
That there may be cases where the physician can
do little more for his patient than to commit him
thus to the wide world, I am not prepared to
deny; but they are rare, I believe; at least, I
did not meet with any such during a residence
of many years on the Continent, where my intercourse with patients of this class was pretty
extensive. On the contrary, a single case did
not fall under my observation, in which minute
and careful examination could not detect a de-

ranged state, either in the functions or the structure of some organ or viscus, the mitigation of which, previous to his journey, would not have contributed to the mental as well as the bodily health of the patient, or in which a proper regimen would not have favoured greatly the effects of climate, and facilitated the recovery. When we are better acquainted with the morbid conditions of the internal organs, and especially of those of the mucous membranes, and with the extensive influence which they exert on the mind, we shall have less frequent occasion to confess our ignorance of the patient's complaints, by attributing them to nervousness, to low spirits, or other imaginary states, designated by like expressions without any definite meaning.

With regard to the general management of these cases while the patient is travelling,—the same directions are applicable as to the more recent cases of dyspepsia, and which have just been detailed.

As on the journey, so during their residence abroad, the diet is the most important circumstance requiring the attention of dyspeptic invalids. Since the stomach is the organ primarily and principally affected, it does not require any argument to prove that, unless the diet be such as is suited to its morbid condition, climate or any other means will do little good. It is impos-

sible, however, in this place, to do more than to
point out the kind of diet which, from experience,
I found most generally suited to this class of
invalids. I have already remarked, and it is a
circumstance that should never be lost sight of
by all classes of travellers, that, in removing to
a warmer climate, the sensibility of the system is
increased, and it is, consequently, more easily
excited by stimulants of every description. Hence,
the diet that may be borne with impunity in
England, will not agree in Italy, nor in the
south of France. This remark is more particularly applicable to persons suffering from stomach
complaints. There is, no doubt, a difference in
dyspeptic patients as well as others in this respect;
but I invariably found a mild and very moderate
diet the most suitable for them; and for this
plain reason,—that whatever may be the nature
of the disorder of the stomach, debility, or, in
other words, a diminution in the powers of the
organ for the performance of its functions is,
with a few rare exceptions, an accompaniment of
the disease.

Wine should always be taken in great moderation; and when this is permitted, it will be
found that the lighter kinds, if not acid, generally
agree the best. Of wines imported into Italy,
those of France are the best, especially sound
claret and sauterne. The spirituous wines of

Spain, Portugal, and Sicily are very injurious. Soda or Seltzer water will often prove a good substitute for wine.

The dessert is a constant source of temptation and mischief in stomach affections, and it would be a wise rule for all dyspeptic patients to abstain entirely from every thing that comes to the table in that form. This advice I feel cannot be urged too strongly. The dyspeptic patient cannot have too forcibly impressed upon him that temperance and abstemiousness are the best physic. The notion so generally entertained that medicine can counteract the effects of habitual errors in regimen, should be regarded as mere sophistry. There is but one road to a permanent cure in these cases, but it is a sure one; and he who shall steadily pursue it long enough to feel its advantages in the restoration of that mental and bodily energy which he had lost, will not easily be induced to deviate from it again.

Exercise in the open air is one of the greatest advantages which a southern climate affords; and the dyspeptic invalid should take the full benefit of it. Walking and horse exercise are the best, but neither should be taken so as to produce much fatigue. When the irritation of the stomach is complicated with that of the bronchial membrane, riding should be chiefly relied on for exercise. Exercising the arms by means of dumb bells, every morning, is very useful in dyspeptic complaints; as are, likewise, reciting and reading aloud. While on the subject of exercise I must not omit to mention that on the water, which to many invalids is very soothing and beneficial, —yacht-sailing is an excellent remedy for dyspepsia, if aided by proper regimen.

Friction of the whole surface, night and morning, is a valuable remedy, and is especially suited to the sedentary, as being the best substitute for exercise. For those whose occupation compels them to a sedentary life, in our own damp and cold climate, there are few remedies more useful, though none more neglected, than friction. The diligent use of this during winter, and sponging the whole surface with cold vinegar and water, or the shower bath, daily, during summer, and the occasional use of the warm bath during spring and autumn, regulated according to the constitution of the patient, form a powerful combination of means for maintaining the health of such persons as are constrained by circumstances to forego the natural modes of bodily exercise in the open air; and the same measures are often singularly efficacious in restoring the diminished energy of the skin and digestive organs in cases of nervous and congestive dyspepsia. These measures, however, should not be considered as superseding exercise in the open air where this is practicable. For the want of this, nothing can fully compensate; but the plan which I have suggested, will enable the system, in some degree, to bear the want of it, and will always prove beneficial, as an additional remedy, in the class of invalids for whom I am now writing.

Cold and damp are particularly injurious in dyspepsia, more especially in the nervous and congestive forms, in which coldness of the surface and extremities, is a prominent symptom. The use of warm clothing, therefore, forms an essential part of the treatment. Flannel should be worn next the skin; and when any change of dress is made in the summer, it should be done gradually and with great caution; and the change of weather in autumn should always be anticipated by a return to warmer clothing. These precautions are equally necessary in a southern climate.

All these measures tend directly to maintain a free circulation through the extremities and surface,—an object which is never to be lost sight of in the treatment of dyspepsia. Indeed I conceive that it is chiefly in consequence of the active circulation on the surface during the warmth of summer, that so many feeble, dyspeptic and nervous invalids find themselves better and get fatter during that season; and that the hypochondriac's mind is freed of half the gloom which oppressed it,—as it is from the decrease of the superficial circulation, and the consequent congestion of the internal viscera, that such

patients languish during nine months of the year
in this country. On this principle, the advantage
of passing the winter in a mild climate may be
partly explained.

If the measures which I have just recommended,
be steadily adhered to, little medicine will be
required. It will at all times be necessary to
attend to the state of the bowels; though the
dyspeptic invalid should endeavour to bring them
to act regularly by proper regimen rather than
by medicine. That this may generally be done,
even in very obstinate cases of constipation, I
am satisfied from experience ; and in young
persons a regular state of bowels may often be
induced, in a much shorter period than could
be believed, after years of suffering from an
opposite state. Generally speaking, the same
advice which I gave on this subject to invalids
while travelling, will apply equally well when they
are stationary.

Medicines which act more directly by allaying
the irritation of the stomach, should only be taken
under medical advice ; as their proper application
to the form and degree of the disease of the
stomach, is a point of too great nicety for the
invalid to decide for himself. A very simple and
one of the best direct remedies in gastric
dyspepsia, in a subdued degree, is a tea spoonful
of castor oil, at bed time occasionally ; and, its
beneficial effects on the stomach have generally

appeared to me more evident when it did not act on the bowels. By allaying the irritation of the stomach, it favours sleep, and diminishes the disposition to morning headach, dry tongue, &c. Water-ices may often be advantageously used in gastritic dyspepsia. These are best taken when the stomach is empty, and should be swallowed slowly; when so used, they will prove cooling and somewhat tonic. Even small portions of solid ice, taken whole into the stomach, often prove a useful tonic in gastritic dyspepsia.

Another simple remedy and one which often proves very useful in the same form of the disease, is a glass of cold water, sipped slowly in the morning when the patient is dressing, provided there is not much disposition to headach or pain of the stomach. Fluids ought to be taken slowly at all times by dyspeptics, that is, sipped rather than drunk. The ancient physicians who observed the good effects of this practice, ordered their patients to drink through a syphon. This would be a good practice to be adopted by many dyspeptics; and if some means could be devised of obliging them to chew their food deliberately and perfectly, a still greater benefit would accrue to this class of persons. Imperfect mastication, indeed, is one of the most common sources of dyspepsia. In old age, when the appetite often continues good and the loss of teeth renders mastication impossible, this is a constant source of gastritic dyspepsia; and in younger persons who lose their teeth early in life, the same thing frequently occurs.

In obstinate disorders of the digestive organs, a course of mineral waters, after a winter passed in a mild climate, will often be of great service. A residence for some time in a proper climate, and a suitable regimen, may have allayed the irritation of the mucous surfaces, and induced a more healthy action in these and in the skin; but something more active may be required to remove the venous congestion of the abdominal organs, and to promote a freer and more steady action of the liver and other glandular viscera connected with digestion. With this view I consider a well applied course of mineral waters, suited to the particular nature of the disease, a very valuable remedy, and capable of effecting in many cases what no other remedy with which I am acquainted can effect. The selection of the mineral water must depend upon the peculiar nature of the derangement and degree of susceptibility of the digestive organs, and upon the secondary disorders which may have been induced in other parts of the system. I can only venture on some general directions here.*

---

* Full information respecting the medical qualities and employment of these waters in disorders of the digestive organs, &c., will be found in a work which I intend publishing immediately on the subject of MINERAL WATERS.

When the mucous surfaces are in a state of irritation, and the liver and abdominal venous

As many persons, in whose complaints these waters are indicated, may find it inconvenient to take a course of them at their sources, it may not be irrelevant to our present subject to say a few words respecting the Artificial Mineral Waters which have lately been introduced into this country by Dr. Struve of Dresden. When in Germany, I made particular inquiries regarding the estimation in which these waters were held by the physicians of the different cities in which Dr. Struve had establishments. The information which I obtained, more especially at Berlin, where these artificial waters are extensively employed, was invariably in favour of their decided utility; and the remarkable similarity in their effects to those of the natural waters was generally admitted. The respectability of Dr. Struve, and his skill as a chemist, were also universally acknowledged.

After such satisfactory information, obtained from physicians of the highest character in Germany, I had no hesitation in prescribing the waters of the German Spa at Brighton in the same cases in which I should have recommended a course of the natural waters of Ems, Carlsbad, &c., had not the distance of these places presented obstacles to their employment. During the last two seasons, I have had sufficient experience of the beneficial effects of Dr. Struve's waters to satisfy me of their decided utility in several of the diseases treated of in this work, more especially in the class of disorders which forms the subject of the present article. And I feel convinced that when their beneficial effects are more generally known to the profession, and the manner of taking them better understood, they will be extensively employed in a numerous class of patients suffering from disorders of the digestive organs, &c. At the same time, I have no hesitation in saying, that if the patient could conveniently take a course of the natural mineral waters at their respective sources, I should decidedly prefer this.

system generally, are in a congested state, or where the functions of the uterus are defective, and there is not much relaxation of the system, the mineral waters of EMS, of VICHY, or of PLOMBIERES, will be useful, particularly the two first. In cases where the skin is in an unhealthy state, or where there is dyspeptic disease complicated with chronic bronchial disease, and no objection exists to an elevated mountainous country, CAUTERETS, among the Pyrenees, will deserve a preference.

When the abdominal viscera are in a more obstinately congested and torpid state, and where there does not exist much irritation of the mucous surfaces, the waters of CARLSBAD will be more useful than any of these. In some cases, a course of the EMS water may precede the use of those of Carlsbad with great advantage. Where more pure nervous debility exists, and there is a degree of atony of the stomach; or when the uterine system is debilitated and relaxed, without there being as yet any organic disease, the cold chalybeate waters of SPA will be useful, and, still more, those of PYRMONT. The internal use of the latter is often combined with a course of warm bathing in the same with excellent effect. But to derive essential benefit from this class of waters, the digestive organs must be free from irritation, and the vascular system not in a state of plethora. For patients labouring under gastritic dyspepsia, who may visit Naples, the aërated sulphureous water of SAN LUCIA will be found beneficial, and may be used in combination with warm sea-bathing very advantageously.

In other cases of stomach disorders, a course of goat's whey at GEISS in Switzerland, or some mountainous situation in our own country, as in Wales or Scotland, may be preferable to mineral waters. This is a practice much employed in some parts of the continent, and, I believe, with considerable success. The cases in which this is more particularly indicated, are the forms of gastritic dyspepsia, in which there is much sensibility, and at the same time a degree of languor in the system, without a very deranged state of the abdominal organs or skin. In young persons in whom the gastric irritation has induced a disposition to convulsions or epilepsy, or in whom a tendency to cerebral congestion exists, threatening hydrocephalus, such a course of whey, and a residence for some time in an elevated mountainous country, will be very useful. The combination of Iceland-moss-jelly with whey, as nutriment, will be often of great service in obstinate cases of gastritic dyspepsia in this class of patients.

In other cases, a course of ripe grapes (*cure de raisins*) will prove very beneficial. Where with a low degree of gastritic dyspepsia, there exists a similar state of the mucous membrane of the intestines, with a disposition to diarrhœa; also in chronic cases of this disease, and in hæmorrhoidal affections, ripe grapes will be of great use in allaying the irritation on which the symptoms depend.

Before concluding the subject of stomach affections, I once more beg that it may be clearly understood that I do not recommend travelling, or a residence in the South of Europe, to patients labouring under the more acute forms of gastritic dyspepsia; much less do I advise such a measure to those labouring under organic disease or chronic inflammation of any of the abdominal viscera. When organic changes have taken place, or inflammation has been established in any organ of importance to life, the case is materially changed from the state which I have had in view. A long journey under such circumstances is more likely to increase than diminish the evil. Whenever inflammation exists in a degree sufficient to influence the action of the heart materially, in whatever organ or structure it may be situated, I consider rest and quiet as most essential parts of the cure, though these are very much neglected in what are, often improperly, called chronic diseases. The diseases in which climate proves most useful are such as depend rather on functional disorder, or in which, if inflammation does exist, it is in a very subdued degree only, and with little disposition to activity. In this case, and when the structures of the different viscera are entire, and the indication is merely to remove functional disease, and to prevent inflammation and its consequences, or to assist the constitution in overcoming the latter, climate may be made a powerful agent.

In bringing to a conclusion this rather extended disquisition on dyspeptic disorders, it may be useful to sum up, under a few heads, the principal results of our inquiries.

1st, Dyspeptic complaints are chiefly referable to, and have their origin in two leading pathological conditions of the stomach,—the one of an inflammatory, the other of a nervous character.

2nd, These two states require two different methods of treatment, and are benefited by climates of a different character; a soft and mild climate, such as that of the south-west of France and of England, being more suitable to the inflammatory form ; and the drier and more exciting climates of the south-east of France and Nice, more beneficial in the nervous and congestive form.

3rd, In complicated cases of dyspepsia, which are the most frequent, the method of treatment, both generally and as regards climate, must be regulated chiefly by the morbid condition which is the more predominant, and which influences the constitution most evidently.   When a secondary series of disorders has been induced, these, as well as the hereditary disposition of the patient, must also be taken into consideration, in selecting a fit climate.

4th, Mineral waters are very valuable remedies in chronic disorders of the digestive organs, and will frequently effect cures after climate and suitable regimen have failed to do more than relieve.

5th, The advantages to be derived from change of air, climate, mineral waters, &c., depend, in a great degree, upon the proper application of these agents to the nature and degree of the disorder, and upon the regimen followed by the patient during their operation.

Finally, No change of climate, or other remedy, can be made permanently beneficial, while the exciting causes of the disease continue to be applied.

CONSUMPTION.

There is no disease in which change of climate is considered in this country of so much importance, as Consumption; and yet it must be admitted, that there is no one in which the hopes founded in such a change, are more constantly disappointed. Occasional examples of its beneficial effects are certainly observed; and, though they bear so trifling a proportion to the cases in which it produces no benefit, or only a temporary and very trifling one, it still remains the chief source of hope and confidence in the treatment of consumption, both to the profession and the public. Nor, when we consider the inefficacy of all other means hitherto adopted to arrest the progress of this disease, need it be matter of surprize that its victims should seek for that relief from a more genial clime, which seems to be denied them in their own. Every one fondly indulges the hope, that he may be the fortunate individual on whom the favourable chance is to fall.

A belief in the efficacy of change of air and climate in consumption, dates from a very early period, and prevails, more or less, at the present day, over the whole civilized world. In this country, indeed, so great is the general confidence in its powers, that the failure is rather attributed to the circumstance of its being had recourse to " too late," than to any want of efficacy in the measure itself. For my own part, although I have witnessed the melancholy issue of too many cases sent abroad at a very early period of the disease, to have much confidence in such a measure singly, still I believe a change to a mild climate, or rather a temporary residence there, to be a valuable remedy, under certain limitations. And I am further of opinion, that when a more rational view of the nature and causes of consumption is generally adopted, change of climate may be made a far more efficient and a more certain remedial agent in that disease, than it has hitherto been.

There is certainly no subject connected with health, which possesses greater claims to the attention of the inhabitants of this country, than that which relates to the causes and nature of that class-of diseases of which consumption is one of the most frequent and fatal forms; at the same time, there is no one concerning which, it appears to me, they are less informed. And it is a matter of still greater regret, that the members of the medical profession are themselves by no means agreed on these points; for until juster views are generally entertained on the subject, not only by them, but by the public at large, we cannot hope to make any sure or steady progress in the prevention of this class of diseases.

Respecting the treatment of consumption, we

must admit the humiliating truth, that there is no reason to believe that the physicians of the present day are more successful than their predecessors were ten, nay twenty centuries ago. Considering, therefore, the vital importance of the subject, how imperfectly it is understood by the public, and what difference of opinion respecting it exists among medical men, I trust no apology may be deemed necessary for occupying a few pages in stating my own views. As the best, therefore, and indeed only means of arriving at clear and satisfactory conclusions concerning it, I shall take a general though brief view of the nature, the causes and progress of consumption; and this will, at the same time, enable me to state, with greater precision, what may reasonably be expected from climate, as a preventive of this disease, and what it promises at the different periods of its progress, and under its different complications.

It is now clearly ascertained by pathologists, that the immediate cause of pulmonary consumption, or that which constitutes its essential character, is the existence, in the lungs, of certain substances called tubercles. As these bodies·form the first evident link in the succession of morbid changes in the lungs, which produce the well known phenomena of consumption, I shall take them as a fixed point from which to commence my present inquiry; it being clear, that in our researches into the nature of consumption, our first object should be to ascertain the origin of tubercles. Until we arrive at a knowledge of the state of the system which leads to the formation of these bodies, and of the causes which induce this state, we cannot hope to establish rules for the prevention of consumption upon any sound principles. I say *prevention* of consumption,— because to cure it even in its earlier stages, in other words, to remove tubercles already existing in the lungs, is what we can scarcely hope to do. "La guérison de la Phthisie tuberculeuse n'est pas au-dessus des forces de la nature ; mais nous devons avouer en même temps que l'art ne possède encore aucun moyen certain d'arriver à ce but."* The utmost, I fear, that we can reasonably expect in the present state of the art, when tubercles are already formed, is to retard their progress, and to prevent their successive formation; and even our best directed efforts in this way are chiefly of a negative kind. Some, indeed, are sanguine enough to believe that tubercles may be absorbed. But of this we have no positive proof; and there is too much reason to fear, that, when once formed, they are little influenced by any remedies hitherto discovered, but advance, with more or less rapidity, through their

---

* Laennec.

different stages, and ultimately terminate in the destruction of that portion of the lungs in which they are imbedded; and which, in a frightful proportion of cases, ends in the destruction of the patient. Yet the expulsion from the lungs, by expectoration, of the softened tuberculous matter, occasionally leads to the permanent cure of the disease; and, in the opinion of some of the best pathologists of the present day, this is the only way in which a cure of tuberculous consumption is effected. But such fortunate cases bear a ratio so extremely small to the number of fatal terminations, that they can hardly be considered as controverting the truth of the position—that tubercles may be prevented, but are scarcely to be cured. I do not by this mean to affirm, that tubercles never are absorbed; on the contrary, I am disposed to believe that they may be so, especially in the young subject. But it must be confessed, that the present state of our knowledge on this subject, as well as the limited powers of our art, lead us to place little reliance on the absorption of tubercles, and should rather excite our exertions (and this I feel most anxious to impress on the minds of my readers) to prevent their formation, by preventing or correcting the condition of the system in which they have their origin.

The next step, therefore, in our researches, leads us to inquire into the proximate cause of

tubercles. Are they a product of inflammation, as
is believed by some pathologists? or, are they the
result of a specific action, totally unconnected
with inflammation, arising out of and depending
upon a morbid condition of the general system, as
is the opinion of others? This is a most important inquiry; as upon the conclusions which we
arrive at respecting it, must depend, in a great
degree, the nature of the measures we adopt for
the prevention of consumption. The formation of
tubercles has been very generally attributed to
inflammation affecting the different structures
which compose the lungs, or the other organs in
which they are deposited. We very frequently
hear it stated that such a person was attacked with
inflammation of the lungs, and which was speedily
followed by consumption. As consumption was
thus generally considered a consequence of
inflammatory affections of the chest, so when
tubercles were found to be the constant proximate
cause of consumption, they were naturally supposed to be the result of inflammation.

But the progress of morbid anatomy and more
minute and more correct observation have discovered, that tubercles may be formed without
even the slightest symptoms of inflammation, and
without any of the usual traces of its existence
being detected; whilst, on the other hand, inflammation in all its degrees is of frequent occurrence without giving rise to tubercles. Nothing is

more common than to find tubercles in numerous
organs of the body at the same time, and it is
often in that organ only in which they had longest
existed, (commonly the lungs,) that traces of
inflammation are to be found,—the tubercles being
frequently deposited in the unchanged, healthy
structure of the part. As striking examples of
this fact, we may cite the existence of tubercles
in the brain of children where no signs of inflammation are to be discovered until, from their size,
they become, as other foreign bodies, sources of
irritation. In the instance, also, of tubercles or
substances closely resembling these, being speedily
produced in the lower animals by want of exercise,
bad food, confined air, and want of light, &c.,
inflammation will scarcely be adduced as a principal cause.

We all know that tubercles are often very in-
sidious in their formation and increase ; and most
pathologists agree that, in a very large proportion
of those cases of colds and inflammatory affections
of the lungs which appear to lay the foundation
of consumption, the tubercles exist previously to
the occurrence of these diseases, although they
may not produce any marked symptoms by which
their presence can be recognized. That tubercles
in any organ should render it more prone to
inflammation, is easily to be conceived ; but
that simple inflammation should be capable of
producing such extensive alterations without its

existence being discoverable during life by any of the usual signs, or any traces of it being detected after death, is a conclusion which it is difficult to admit.

Whilst the foregoing facts and observations induce us to believe that tubercles are not generally the result of inflammation, it cannot be doubted, on the other hand, that there are instances in which tubercles are more immediately connected with this pathological state. Now, admitting this, whence does it arise that the same morbid action gives origin to tubercles in one instance and not in the other? If tubercles are simply the result of inflammation, how comes it that inflammation, so frequent an occurrence, is so seldom found to leave traces of tubercles? It is obvious that, in order that tubercles should be the result of inflammation, there must be some modified condition of the inflammation; and if we inquire more closely we shall find that another disorder is connected with the inflammation, and that this disorder is the essential agent in the production of tubercles. In a healthy subject, I believe tubercles are never the result of inflammation. When, therefore, these appear to be the product of inflammation, it will be found to be inflammation occurring in and modified by a disordered state of the system of a peculiar kind. And, surely, it is more reasonable to attribute the tubercles to this chachectic state, which is almost constantly observed, than to the inflammation which is only occasionally detected, and which, in innumerable instances, is found to be of itself insufficient for their production.

To this disordered state of the system it behoves the physician to direct his chief attention. It is only by correcting it that he can prevent the formation of tubercles, or, in other words, prevent consumption.

I do not mean by these remarks to underrate the injurious effects of pulmonary inflammation in persons disposed to consumption, or already labouring under its early symptoms ; on the contrary, I am fully sensible of the great importance of preventing inflammation, and of removing it when it has occurred in such subjects. And, although I do not consider inflammation as the cause of tubercles, I agree with most pathologists in believing that it accelerates their progress. It certainly renders the disease more complicated, more difficult of management, and more rapidly fatal. What I object to is the opinion which regards inflammation as the source of all the evil, and considers the removal of it as the only or principal means of preventing the further progress of the disease.

Although I have adopted these views after careful observation, and unbiassed by the opinions of others, I do not wish them to be considered as peculiar to me. They are in accordance, I believe, with those of some of the best pathologists of the day, both English and foreign.

In some cases, as I have already observed, the phenomena which accompany, or seem to indicate the developement of tubercles, certainly lead to the belief that inflammation, or, at least, some increase of vascular action, is connected with their formation; and, in other instances, the inflammatory exudation forms evidently the nidus in which tubercles are deposited, as is often distinctly seen in cases of peritoneal inflammation. But this occurs only, I believe, in the unhealthy subject. In a still greater number of cases, simple congestion of the lungs appears to be connected with the origin of tubercles, and is probably even necessary for their formation.

The immediate process by which tubercles are produced is involved in much obscurity. It may be a peculiar action of the extreme vessels totally unconnected with inflammation or even increased action, at least, we have no proof that any such increased action takes place. Their formation is just as likely, for any thing we know to the contrary, to be the result of a morbid diminution of action,—a supposition, by the way, which the pathological phenomena observed in many consumptive subjects seem rather to support. The vessels of any organ may deposit the matter of tubercle in the place of that which should be secreted to maintain the healthy organization of the body; such deviation from the natural action depending, probably, as well on the morbid state of the fluids, as on a depraved action of the vessels, both originating in a cachectic state of the system generally.*

* Amidst the discrepancy of opinions which exists on this obscure subject, I have much pleasure in giving the views of my ingenious friend, Dr. Todd, with which, at my request, he has favoured me, and which, it will be seen, are in accordance with my own.

" The opinion which I entertain of the nature of tubercles and of the manner in which they are formed is, that they are depositions of coagulable lymph of a deficient degree of vitality, produced by a peculiar depravation of the function of assimilation, the consequence of a general disorder of the constitution. But, how any aberration in the function of assimilation should lead to the deposition of coagulable lymph, and how tubercles should be the result of such depositions, are points which require further explanation.

" Physiologists are now disposed to believe, that in the function of nutrition, the constituent particles of each particular structure are not directly secreted or deposited by the nutrient vessels, but that there is an intermediate or previous process, which is the deposition of the peculiar matter well known under the name of coagulable lymph. They find proofs of this intricate process in the growth and developement of the embryo, in the formation and growth of the chick *in ovo*, in the process by which, in the more perfect animals, breaches of continuity are united and lost parts restored, and entire members regenerated, in the lower ones. Of this account of nutrition the following extract from a paper on the process of reproduction of the members of the lower animals will, perhaps, afford some additional illustration.

" ' The process of growth naturally leads us to consider the more general law of organization, from which it would seem to emanate. I mean the formation of structures or tissues through the intermediate agency of that substance which we call coagu-

It seems probable that inflammation occurring under such circumstances, may lead to the formation of tubercles; and it will certainly be an additional source of irritation in the lungs and to lable lymph. Indeed, it would seem that this substance is the matrix of every structure. It is the simplest form of animal existence, and it is the first form of existence of even the most perfect animals. It is the medium through which every breach of continuity is united, and by which every loss of substance is restored, and although it is only on such occasions that its existence and importance are known to us, there is good reason to believe, that it exists constantly as a separate and independent part in all animals in a greater or less degree, and that it is through its means that the whole process of nutrition is carried on.

" ' Coagulable lymph is decidedly possessed of a principle of vitality and in its healthy state is capable of organization. It is most particularly distinguished by its power of forming blood vessels. These vessels are entirely independent of those already existing, but they afterwards become united to and continuous with them. Nor does any other source but this substance present itself for the first formation of the blood in the chick in ovo.'*

" If the above statement be a correct account of the function of nutrition, it must be readily understood how this lymph, deficient in the usual degree of vitality, and, hence, incapable of organization, instead of becoming the natural structure of a part, may give rise to tubercles, under every form and variety in which they present themselves, and also, how coagulable lymph of such an imperfect nature, should be a consequence of a general state of cachexy of the body.

" Nor does this opinion of the formation of tubercles exclude

* On the Process of Reproduction of the Members of the Aquatic Salamander, by T. I. Todd.—*Journal of the Royal Institution.*

the constitution generally. In persons strongly predisposed to tubercular disease, the frequent occurrence of catarrh or of pulmonary inflammation, may, by keeping up a degree of con-

the possibility of their being also, indirectly, the result of inflammation; for I believe I am not peculiar in regarding the process of nutrition and the adhesive inflammation as only different degrees or forms of the same function. On the contrary, I am disposed to believe that the formation of tubercles after inflammation affords both a proof and an illustration of my opinion.

" With this view, I will cite the example of tubercles formed in new growths, the products of inflammation, as in the false membranes of tubercular peritonitis. Now this we know affords us, in the first place, a proof of tubercles being formed from coagulable lymph, and if, in the second place, we inquire why the organization of the new growth is not perfected, but has deviated from its natural course, and given rise to tubercles, we shall find that there is some condition superadded or combined with the inflammation. The histories of this disease explain what is the nature of this condition and show that it almost universally occurs in disordered, unhealthy subjects, where all the functions are imperfectly performed. So that even here when these tubercles appear to be the result of inflammation, if the circumstances be more closely analyzed, it appears that inflammation is not a direct cause of them, but only indirectly so, as affording the substance or materials for their production. The essential cause is the unhealthy nature of the lymph, the effects of a general cachectic state of the body.

" Nor is this inquiry mere matter of speculative curiosity, for, if the views which I have taken of this morbid process be well founded, they ought to lead to important practical results, as tending to fix the attention more steadily on the origin of the disease, the only possible way which can lead to its prevention.

" *Brighton, April 25th,* 1829.　　　　　T. I. Todd."

gestion and irritation of the lungs, give rise to the formation of tubercles at an earlier period than would otherwise have happened, and may even, in nicely balanced cases, determine their occurrence: or, to express myself more clearly, I believe that in a system labouring under tubercular cachexy, tubercles may be the product of a low degree of inflammation. But in these cases the tubercles cannot fairly be considered the simple product of inflammation; it merely acts upon a deranged state of system as an exciting and occasional cause.

The real cause of tubercles, I believe, with Dr. Todd and some other pathologists, to be a morbid condition of the general system, hereditary in some, but induced in others, and increased, in all cases, by a series of functional derangements ultimately affecting the whole animal economy. This state of the system may be denominated *Tubercular Cachexy*.

I proceed to point out some of the leading symptoms by which this state is characterized; but I must be allowed to premise that it is more easily recognized than described: for this affection being a progressive one, the signs by which it is characterized are more or less manifest according to the degree in which it exists.

The appearance of the countenance of a patient labouring under this disorder, is one of the first circumstances which attracts observation. If the expression of the features is indicative of mental feelings, it is equally so of the physical condition of the internal organs; upon their integrity depends mainly the healthy character of the countenance. In the affection we are now considering, it is generally paler than natural, though at different times, and without any apparent reason, it is in this respect subject to striking changes. Where there is naturally much colour, these changes are often very remarkable. At one time there is a general paleness, with a sunk, faded appearance of the countenance; at another, an irregular mixture of white and red. In place of the natural gradations by which these colours pass into each other in health, they terminate by distinct and abrupt lines, giving the face a blotched or spotted appearance. Sallow complexions assume a peculiarly unhealthy aspect, exhibiting a dull, leaden hue, diffused over a general palid ground : there is also paleness of the lips. The eyes have generally a pearly, glassy appearance, and the whole countenance has commonly a sunk and languid aspect. But these appearances, as I have already said, are very variable. They are at first also transitory, and often pass unnoticed, except by the eye of an anxious parent or by the physician; but as the system feels more strongly the influence of the tubercular disorder, they become evident to the most cursory observer. Before putting a question to such a patient, the physician who has been accustomed to trace the progress of the morbid condition under consideration, to mark the changes which the countenance assumes under it, and to connect these with the general disorder, knows full well what replies will follow his inquiries.

Upon closer examination, the skin of such a patient will be found in an unhealthy condition. It will be either harsh and dry, or this state will be found to alternate with a moist, clammy, and relaxed one. Its colour, too, is often changed to a sallow, and, in some cases, to a dirty yellowish hue; and, except on the cheeks, there is always a deficiency of red vessels. In some hereditary cases, particularly in females of a fair and delicate complexion, the skin assumes a semi-transparent appearance, resembling wax-work, and the veins may be seen distinctly through it. The temperature, also, of the surface and extremities, will generally be found to be below the standard of health.

In tubercular cachexy, the digestive organs are very generally more or less deranged, though the degree and nature of the derangement differ materially in different cases. The tongue is generally more or less furred, especially towards the base ; the extremity and edges are in some cases pale and flabby ; in others, with the furred base, the point and margin are redder than natural,

and often studded with enlarged papillæ of a
still brighter hue : these are also frequently seen
projecting through the fur which is spread over
its central and back parts. The former state
of the tongue is a more frequent accompaniment
of that form of the disease which originates
chiefly in hereditary predisposition ; the latter,
of that which is principally or entirely acquired,
and in which an irritated state of the stomach
attends the disorder from the beginning and often
preceeds it. In both cases, the functions of the
digestive organs are badly performed. In a third
class of cases, of much rarer occurrence, the
tongue is clean and natural in its appearance,
and the digestive organs perform their functions
pretty regularly. I have, I think, remarked this
chiefly in females, in whom the disease has been
mainly owing to hereditary predisposition, and
has been little complicated with gastric irritation.
In the same manner as the state of the tongue,
so do the functions of the stomach and bowels
vary. In the last case, the appetite and digestion
are generally good, and the bowels pretty regular ;
and the individual bears and even requires a
stronger and fuller diet. But, in the other cases,
the functions of the digestive organs are more or
less deranged, the appetite being irregular, often
capricious, the digestion imperfect, the bowels
more or less constipated, and the alvine eva-
cuations indicating an unhealthy state of the

biliary and intestinal secretions. The urine varies; it is generally high coloured and charged with sediment; very generally also it is covered with an oily or irridescent pellicle. But the state of the urine is greatly dependant upon that of the digestive organs and skin.

The state of the circulation is subject to great variety. In hereditary cases, I think the powers of the heart are commonly under the ordinary standard, whilst the frequency of the pulse is generally above it, and palpitation is not an unfrequent symptom. The circulation is in general imperfectly carried on through the extreme vessels, as is shown by the condition of the skin already noticed, and the tendency to coldness of the extremities. This state of the surface and extremities is a very constant attendant on a congested and embarrassed state of the abdominal vessels, complicated with an irritated condition of the mucous surfaces; and hence it is generally more evident, according as the disorder of the digestive organs is more considerable. The general strength is diminished. This is an early symptom, more especially in females, and is shown by the patient's gait and motions, which are indicative of languor and debility: there is a disinclination for exercise, particularly in the early part of the day, and, on examination, the muscles will be found to have lost their tone, and to have become soft and relaxed.

The nervous system also partakes in the early derangements. There is more nervous sensibility than is natural to the patient. The sleep is not sound, being disturbed or unnaturally heavy, and rarely refreshing. The mind sympathizes with the bodily disorder, and loses its natural energy. The temper also is often remarkably changed. In the purer and less complicated cases of hereditary consumption, there is generally great serenity of mind; the spirits are often of surprising buoyancy, when compared with the state of the body; and hope mingles its cheering influence almost with the last sufferings of the patient. But this state of mind is a less constant attendant on consumption than is generally believed; especially in those cases in which disorder of the digestive organs leads to the morbid condition of the system, which terminates in tubercular cachexy.

The symptoms which I have just enumerated as characteristic of the deranged state of the constitution, which precedes consumption, and which I have denominated Tubercular Cachexy, vary considerably. Some are more or less remarkable in different cases, though they may, I believe, be observed in by far the greater number of such patients, during a longer or shorter period, before the occurrence of symptoms which indicate the existence of pulmonary disease.

Under the general term, consumption, then, we may comprehend three different forms or stages of disease—1st, general disorder of the health; 2nd, tubercular cachexy; 3rd, consumption, properly so called. These different stages may, in general, be distinctly recognized; though it is only in proportion to the physician's powers and habits of minute and careful observation, that the symptoms of the first stage will be remarked, or, in other words, that he will be able to detect the approach of the confirmed tubercular disease.

In persons with a strong hereditary taint, the first stage is less easily observed, because, in truth, it may be said to be their natural state. On the other hand, in those cases where the predisposition is acquired, the degree of constitutional disorder which precedes and accompanies consumption in its progress is more apparent, and exists for a longer period before the tubercular state is fully formed. Consumption in such cases generally occurs, also, at a later period of life, and is generally slower in its course. In the children of weak, dyspeptic parents the disorder of the general health is very observeable, but in those of consumptive parents, where such a condition of the system is coeval with their birth, it is much less so.

Cases now and then do occur, and the subjects according to my observation, are chiefly delicate young females, in whom tubercular disease steals on so imperceptibly, or is indicated by such faint signs that the patient is on the very brink of the

grave, before the friends are aware of the existence
of danger; but this is a rare case, and will be
still more so, as the state of such patients is more
minutely investigated.

Among the causes of the constitutional disorder
which precedes and leads to consumption, and of
which I have endeavoured to point out the usual
signs, the hereditary nature of the disease requires
our first notice.

The hereditary origin of consumption is too
evident in many cases to be contested; yet it
is equally true that we frequently meet with the
disease in persons in whom no hereditary taint can
be traced. Before proceeding further, it may be
well to state the precise meaning which I attach
to the expression *hereditary predisposition,* as there
has been some confusion in the application of this
term, as well as that of hereditary disease. By
hereditary predisposition, I understand a peculiar
condition of the system, depending upon its original conformation and organization, and derived
from the parents, which renders the individual
more susceptible of, or more liable to lapse into,
certain diseases, than other persons endowed
originally with a more healthy organization. It
is in this way only that consumption can be said
to be hereditary. The child of consumptive
parents is more liable to consumption in its
progress to maturity, than a child whose parents

are perfectly healthy; and unless the condition of the system which constitutes this hereditary predisposition be corrected by proper management in early life, the individual will very probably fall a victim to consumption, or some of those diseases, which, having a close affinity to it, originate in the same state of constitution. It does not follow, however, as a necessary consequence, that a child, who is born with a predisposition to a disease, must be attacked with that disease; all that our observation enables us to affirm is, that the disease in question will be more easily induced in such a person than in another exempt from the same predisposition. It is true that the hereditary predisposition to consumption seems so strong in some individuals and families, that, without any cognizable cause, the regular actions of the economy become deranged, and the system falls into the morbid state which terminates eventually in consumption : Nay, in some rare instances, the infant at birth has been found to be labouring under tubercular disease. On the other hand, so weak is the predisposition in many individuals, that a combination of powerful causes long applied is scarcely adequate to induce the disease. Between these two extremes there exists every variety of shade in the disposition to consumption.

There is another way in which a disposition to consumption and scrofula is transmitted from parents to their children, viz., by the deteriorating influence of other diseases in the parents on the physical condition of their offspring. The children of dyspeptic, of gouty, and of cachectic parents, for example, are very liable to scrofula and consumption ; and this, though a more remote, is probably the original source of scrofulous and tuberculous diseases.

But, as I have already stated, the predisposition to consumption is very often acquired without any hereditary taint ; that is, the tubercular diathesis is induced by the operation of external or accidental causes,—of which this is the proper place to take some notice. To go into detail, however, on this subject, although I admit it to be the most important part of the whole inquiry connected with consumption, would carry me far beyond the limits necessarily prescribed to this work. I shall, therefore, only take a brief and very general view of what appears to me to be the leading causes, in order that this article may be less imperfect than it otherwise would be. I may remark, in passing, that no person, however healthful may have been his original organization, no age, no condition of life, can be considered totally exempt from the liability to consumption : it is met with in early infancy, and occasionally proves fatal to the octogenarian.

Generally speaking, all causes which lower the tone of the bodily health predispose to consumption. Of this kind are,—sedentary occupations, especially in confined and obscure places, a residence in large towns and cities, or in low humid and cold situations, unwholesome or improper diet, imperfect clothing, and long continued functional disease of most organs, but more especially and more frequently of the digestive organs. The abuse of strong spirituous or fermented liquors, especially when added to the preceding causes, I believe very often induces, and certainly hurries on, tubercular disease. All diseases which induce what is called " a bad habit of body," and every kind of debility from accidental causes, predispose to consumption. The frequent occurrence of symptoms of consumption in young persons, soon after they have suffered from severe diseases or long confinement, is matter of frequent observation. Hence the necessity of attention, particularly in delicate subjects, during the convalescence from acute diseases, by which the physical powers have been lowered, and the susceptibility increased. And this attention should be still greater when any local irritation is a sequela of the disease, such as generally occurs in the mucous membranes of the chest or digestive organs after measles, small pox, hooping cough, and scarlatina. To unsuitable diet, exposure to cold, over-fatigue, or resuming too early their usual avocations during convalescence from these diseases, as far as my observation goes, is generally to be attributed the fatal train of morbid phenomena which so often succeed them. The influence of depressing passions must not be omitted among the predisposing causes. They are considered by Morton, Laennec, and some others, the most frequent of all the causes of consumption. Mental depression operating on a constitution already predisposed to tubercular disease, is, without doubt, one of the most certain means of accelerating the evil, and it is in such constitutions that the destructive influence of mental despondency is most conspicuous.

These causes may commence their operation at any period of life, but the origin of the constitutional disorder which I have described as leading ultimately to consumption, is very often to be traced to the mismanagement of children. The seeds of disease, which are to ripen at a later period of life, are frequently sown during infancy and childhood,—in the first case by imperfect suckling, or the entire substitution of artificial food for the natural and only proper nourishment of infants; and in the second, by improper and often over-stimulating food; by a residence in large towns, and in confined, overheated apartments; by deficient exercise in the open air; imperfect clothing, &c.

Girls suffer more especially from some of these causes, such as confinement to the house, often in close rooms; from sedentary occupations; too short and insufficient exercise in the open air, and too much mental application. The first consequences of these are—diminished circulation through the surface and extremities, imperfect digestion and assimilation, a constipated state of bowels, and a congested state of the internal, especially of the abdominal blood vessels, and, very generally, an irritated state of the digestive organs. Then follow, an unhealthy condition of surface, a dry harsh state of the skin generally, cutaneous eruptions, and a disposition to chilblains, sore eyes, glandular swellings, and often curved spine. The appearance of this last symptom is frequently the first thing which excites the alarm of parents, who, in place of directing their attention to the real cause, too often consider the alteration in the shape as the great and primary evil ; and back boards, lying on horizontal planes, and a variety of other mechanical remedies are had recourse to, which not unfrequently add to the mischief, by still further deranging the general health. When the disorder has not gone too far, all that will, in general, be necessary in such cases, is to place the child in circumstances the very reverse of those to which it has been accustomed. Let her be removed to some healthy part of the country, where she can enjoy, free from the injudicious restraints of boarding schools, abundant exercise in the open air, a plain nutritious diet, and have only moderate mental occupation ; and these affections will generally disappear with the return of a healthy condition of the system, of the deterioration of which they were only a consequence. The power of muscular exercise in remedying simple curvatures of the spine, to which I allude, and which arise chiefly from debility and imperfect exercise of the muscles of the trunk, is now pretty well understood ; * but it is not so generally known, that the exercises which are usually employed with this view, though they may strengthen a certain class of muscles, do little for the general health. The exercise which is to benefit the system generally, must be in the open air, and extend to the whole muscular system. If the general health is not restored, the removal of the curvature will avail little ; and, not unfrequently, when the back is improving by daily and long-continued action of its muscles, the general health is becoming worse, as indicated by a pasty, sallow complexion, coarse skin, sore eyes and ears, costive bowels, tumid abdomen, fetid breath, cold extremities, &c. The house exercises now in fashion, and which have been dignified with fine names, are certainly a degree better, if directed with judgment, than the immoveable positions in

---

* For some judicious remarks relative to the state of the muscles of the back, in these cases, and the best mode of treatment, I beg to refer the reader to Dr. Dod's "*Pathological Observations on the Rotated and Contorted Spine.*"

which girls were formerly kept; but if they are
to be made a substitute for exercise in the open
air, they will prove highly injurious to the rising
race of females.   Without regular exercise out
of doors, no young person can continue long
healthy; and it is the duty of parents in fixing
their children at boarding schools (I allude particularly to female children) to ascertain that
sufficient time is occupied daily in this way.   They
may be assured that attention to this circumstance
is quite as essential to the moral and the physical
health of their children, as any branch of education which they may be taught.

The same system of confinement, arising from
an over anxiety to cultivate the mind, is not unfrequently continued during that important period
of life when the system is acquiring its full developement, and a new series of actions is coming
into play; and it is in this case often productive of
incalculable mischief.   It is about the same period
too, when great attention is necessary to maintain
the general health, that the habits of fashionable
life prove most injurious, more especially to females of a delicate constitution.   A few months of
dissipation often turn the scale.   The constitution
which, under more favourable circumstances, might
have been able to maintain a healthy state of
the various functions during this critical period, is
often too weak to resist the destructive influence
of fashionable habits in large towns; and a train

of disorders is thereby induced which destroy the balance of the circulation, and break up the health. In this manner, many individuals are, in a few short months, placed beyond the resources of our art, who, by different management, might have been saved. Or if they do escape, it is often but to exist in a kind of middle state, ever vacillating between health and disease; and, should they become mothers, they will most probably bring into the world only feeble, unhealthy children, prone to the very disease which they themselves have but escaped for a time,—and escaped only perhaps by giving them birth.

It matters little, as to the result, in what organ the mischief begins. The first inroads upon the health, however, are generally made through the organs occupied or immediately connected with the supply and waste of the system,—those organs which perform the important function of digestion and assimilation, and those whose more obvious office is to remove the effete and waste matter from the system. Thus the digestive organs and the skin generally exhibit the earliest symptoms of disorder; and in these, in a very large proportion of cases, may be observed the first links of the chain of morbid actions which undermine the general health and ultimately end in tubercular cachexy.

Though the importance of this subject has already carried me beyond the limits assigned to this article, I cannot resist the opportunity

which the present occasion affords, of stating my
conviction, that it is only by adopting a proper
system of management from the earliest periods
of life that the influence of hereditary predisposition to consumption is to be counteracted,
and a more healthy condition of the body induced.
The stronger the hereditary predisposition is
known to be, or the more delicate the child,
the greater will be the necessity for using every
endeavour to maintain a healthy condition of the
various functions. One of the principal means
of effecting this, is attention to the nature of
the diet, respecting which it appears to me that
very erroneous notions are entertained. The
object should be to afford, in each individual case,
a supply of food suitable as well in quality as
in quantity to the state of the system in general,
but more especially to the powers of the digestive
organs. Upon this subject no general rules can
be laid down that do not admit of numerous
exceptions. Some children require a fuller, some
a medium diet; and others, again, thrive best
on a spare diet. The more common error is
to give children too exciting food, and in too
great quantity. The crude notions that all
scrofulous complaints have their origin in debility,
and are only to be corrected by stimulating, or
what is called nourishing, tonic, or bracing diet,
have now prevailed for such a length of time
as to have grown into a vulgar prejudice. The

consequence of which is, that the tone of the stomach is often destroyed, and the system oppressed and irritated by the very means which are intended to restore it. It seems to be overlooked by the advocates of this plan, that the digestive organs are, in such cases, as weak as any other part of the body,—very often the weakest; and yet they are expected to be the efficient organs of supply for the general system, whilst, at the same time, they are irritated and exhausted by medicines for its relief under every form of disease.

In the earlier periods of life, this over exciting diet, with the purgative system to which it leads, is a fruitful source of disease. The effect of such a diet on delicate children is to produce irritation of mind, a general feverish state, a dry skin, often alternating with copious perspirations, cutaneous eruptions, inflamed eyes, swellings of the lymphatic glands, a disposition to inflammatory diseases, often of a bad character, to fevers, hydrocephalus, &c. To relieve most of these symptoms, recourse is had to the frequent repetition of calomel and other purgatives. Thus the digestive organs, over excited at one time by unsuitable food, and irritated and weakened by purgatives at another, are often permanently injured. The stomach affections, which are so distressing in future life, originate, I am convinced, in many instances, in this method of managing children. It should be kept constantly

in mind, that that kind of food is the best,
which is most adapted to the powers of the
digestive organs, and from which they can most
easily appropriate nourishment suitable to the
system. It is not by the most nutritious food,
but by that which is fitted to the digestive organs,
to the age and susceptibility of the individual,
that the body can be properly nourished or maintained in a state of health. Hence may be
explained the apparently contradictory reports
and opinions which are daily heard respecting the
effects of different kinds of food on delicate and
strumous children,—some affirming that a rich
and highly nutritious diet is proper in all cases ;
others, as strongly contending for a spare and
vegetable one ; each party bringing forward un-
questionable examples of the good effects of their
regimen. To the physician who has attended
to the state of the digestive organs in delicate
and scrofulous children, and to the effects of
different kinds of diet on these organs, and on
the system generally, the explanation of such
cases presents little difficulty.

Living in the country in a healthy situation,
proper clothing, and exercise in the open air, are
the circumstances which next require attention,
as the means of keeping up the tone of the
general health, of maintaining an equable circulation through the body and a healthy condition
of the digestive organs, and of the external and

internal surfaces.* When any derangement of the functions of these organs takes place, it is of the greatest consequence that it should be speedily corrected : for, I regard a diminished circulation through the surface and extremities, and, consequently, a loaded state of the internal, and especially of the abdominal blood vessels, with an irritated state of the mucous surfaces of the stomach and bowels, as constituting, very generally, the first of a series of morbid changes which ultimately end in tubercular cachexy. This in children often takes place with great rapidity. Whether such a state may terminate in disease of the mesenteric glands, of the joints, of the bones, of the spine, or of the lungs or other internal viscera, will depend

---

* As an illustration of these views respecting the influence of air and diet on young subjects disposed to scrofula, the following striking case is given by Bordeu. The child of a peasant at Barèges, a celebrated watering place among the higher Pyrenees, attracted the attention of the visitors, from its fine appearance and quickness, especially of a Princess, who took the child under her care. Previously to this, the child slept upon the grass in common with the sheep, its food being of the coarsest quality, its drink a little whey, often sour. It was now placed in very different circumstances, was fed and clothed and attended to with the greatest care ; but, from change of diet and want of its mountain air, the child soon began to droop ; the mesanterice glands became diseased, and general scrofula declared itself : it died in less than a year. When taken by the Princess it was more healthy and vigorous than its elder brothers, who continued to enjoy health among the mountains, though the whole family were disposed to scrofula.—*Œuvres*, T. I., *p.* 452.

upon the nature of the exciting causes, the age, and numerous other circumstances connected with the peculiarities of structure or form of the individuals. Such, I am satisfied, is the true origin of the numerous train of diseases which I have alluded to, and of consumption the most distressing of all; and this view of the matter cannot, I am convinced, be too strongly impressed upon the minds of parents.

From the frequently hereditary nature of consumption, the death of a parent or one of the family, by this disease, should be a signal for adopting, without delay, the necessary measures to prevent the remaining members of the family from falling victims to it. Supineness under such circumstances may lead to the loss of the whole family. It is useless, in the present state of our knowledge, to talk of curing consumption, seeing that in such a vast proportion of cases, it resists every method of treatment; and from its very nature, I fear it is likely ever to do so, when fully established. Our measures should, therefore, be early and strenuously directed to prevent the disease, by preventing the disordered state of the health, on which it depends, or by correcting this state, if it already exists, whether hereditary or acquired. To do this effectually in cases of strong hereditary predisposition, we must begin with the birth of the infant and not relax our efforts till after the complete developement of the body.

For the removal of the deranged state of the health which we have just been considering, a change to a milder climate is a very powerful remedy, when aided by such other means as the peculiar circumstances of the case may require. Before making such a change, however, the functions of the organs more evidently deranged should, as far as possible, be restored to a healthy state. In a large proportion of cases, the digestive organs and skin, as I have repeatedly remarked, will be found to be disordered, and, until their condition is improved, we shall make no progress in remedying the constitutional disease. But the means employed must be directed with judgment and moderation, as well as steadily persevered in. Violent or very active remedies are not necessary in such cases, but on the contrary, will be injurious. It must be recollected that we have to deal with a constitution either hereditarily weak, or which has been brought into its present condition by a long series of morbid actions, and cannot be at once forced into a healthy state. Even when inflammation exists, we must keep in mind that it is inflammation in a disordered habit, and apply our remedies accordingly. For if the strength is now broken up, and the balance of the circulation suddenly disturbed by debilitating remedies, the system may lapse rapidly into a state of confirmed tubercular cachexy. On the other hand, stimu-

lating or irritating remedies will be equally
pernicious. In the cases now under consideration,
local congestion and irritation are often combined
with general debility; and it requires more judgment to manage this pathological state, than almost
any other with which I am acquainted. The principal object, in such cases, is to promote a more
free and regular distribution of the circulating
fluids through the parts in which they have been
deficient, and to relieve those parts or organs
which have been overloaded. This will be best
done by a mild, nutritious diet suited to the state
of the digestive organs; by exercise in the open
air, especially on horseback, proportioned to the
strength of the patient; by the use of the warm
bath; by cold sponging daily, and friction of the
surface, especially on the chest and extremities.
The removal of gastric or bronchial irritation,
when it exists, and the regulation of the bowels,
are the circumstances which chiefly require the
employment of medicines. The proper application
of these in each individual case, must depend on
the judgment of the medical attendant.

After the disordered functions of the body have
been corrected, the sooner the patient removes to
a mild climate, especially if winter is approaching,
the greater benefit may be expected from the
measure. But this must not be trusted to alone.
On the contrary, the great utility of a removal to

a warm climate, consists in its enabling us to continue the restorative system through the whole year.

Unfortunately it too often happens that the period of functional disease, which we have just been considering, is permitted to pass, before either the patient or his friends are sufficiently aware of the danger. It is not in general till symptoms of irritation or impeded function in the lungs appear, such as cough, shortness of breathing, pain or tightness of the chest, or spitting of blood, that the relations are alarmed, or that fears are expressed that the chest is "threatened." Such symptoms are, alas, too sure indications that tubercular disease is already established in the lungs. It may, indeed, be difficult in many cases to ascertain its positive existence, though, probably, by an attentive consideration of all the circumstances of the case, we shall not err far in our diagnosis; and it need not, at any rate, affect our practice, as a strong suspicion of the presence of tubercles should lead us to adopt the same precautions, as the certainty of their existence.

When tubercles are formed, the circumstances of the patient are materially changed. We have the same functional disorders to remedy which existed in the former state; but we have also organic disease, predisposing to a new series of morbid actions,—to catarrhal affections, hæmoptysis, inflammation of the pleura, &c., which call for important modifications in the plan of treatment. Removal to a mild climate, especially if effected by means of a sea voyage under favourable circumstances, may still be useful, on the same principle as in the former case,—namely, as a means of improving the general health, and of preventing inflammatory affections of the lungs and bronchia. We have seen that the present state of our knowledge on the subject, does not warrant us in placing any reliance on the resolution of tubercles.* That they may remain stationary, and, when not very numerous, be productive of little inconvenience for an unlimited period, is very probable: that they occasionally pass through the various stages of maturation,

---

* With a view of promoting the absorption of tubercles, various medicines have been proposed, and amongst others, *Iodine.* That this medicine may not be useful in this way, as it is in scrofulous affections of other parts of the body, I cannot venture to affirm; but I am quite sure, unless it is employed with much more caution and judgment, and with much more regard to the state of the digestive organs and nervous system, than it has hitherto been, in this country, it is much more likely to prove injurious than useful. I am satisfied it has been productive of very considerable mischief, from the inconsiderate and rash manner in which it has been used. I speak from attentive observation of the effects of this remedy, in cases of Goitre, &c., when employed with much circumspection; and from the numerous examples of its injurious effects, which have come to my knowledge since my return to England.

accompanied with the symptoms of consumption, and that in this way they may ultimately be thrown off by expectoration, and a cure effected, has been demonstrated beyond the possibility of doubt, by Laennec, and other pathologists.* The knowledge, therefore, that tubercles do exist in the lungs should not induce us to relax in our efforts to restore the general health. With this view, a residence in a mild and equable climate, is doubtless one of the most favourable measures which can be adopted, especially if prolonged for several years.

When consumption is fully established,—that is, when the character of the cough and expectoration,

---

* I cannot resist the opportunity here afforded me of recommending to my younger professional brethren, the study of Laennec's valuable work on diseases of the chest, rendered still more valuable in the accurate translation of Dr. Forbes, by the excellent practical notes added to it. Besides indicating a much more certain method of diagnosis of these diseases than we before possessed, this work contains the fullest and clearest account of the pathology of pulmonary diseases, which has ever appeared, and ought to be in the hands of every medical practitioner. On the pathology of Phthisis the work of Louis is excellent; and on the subject of tubercles I may refer the reader to an ingenious "Essai sur les Tubercles," by Dr. H. C. Lombard, of Geneva, the result of whose more extended researches on the same subject, has lately obtained for the author a gold medal, from the Royal Academy of Medicine of Paris, and will, I hope, soon be laid before the public.

the hectic fever and emaciation give every reason
to believe the existence of tuberculous cavities in
the lungs, and, still more, when the presence of
these is ascertained by auscultation,—benefit is
not to be expected from change of climate; and
a long journey will almost certainly increase the
sufferings of the patient, and hurry on the
fatal termination. Under such circumstances, the
patient and his advisers will, therefore, act more
judiciously by contenting themselves with the most
favourable residence which their own country
affords, or even by awaiting the result amid the
comforts of home and the watchful care of friends.
And this will be the more necessary, as the degree
of sympathetic fever and the disposition to inflammation of the lungs or to hæmoptysis is more
considerable.

It is natural for the relations of such a patient
to cling to that which seems to afford even a ray
of hope. But did they know the discomforts,
the fatigue, the exposure and irritation necessarily
attendant on a long journey in the advanced period of consumption, they would shrink from
such a measure. The medical adviser, also, when
he reflects upon the accidents to which such a
patient is liable, will surely hesitate ere he con-
demns him to the additional evil of expatriation.
And his motives for hesitation will be increased
when he considers how often the unfortunate
patient sinks a prey to his disease long before

he reaches the place of destination, or, at best, arrives there in a worse condition than when he left England,—doomed shortly to add another name to the long and melancholy list of his countrymen that have sought with pain and suffering a distant country, only to find in it an untimely grave. When the patient is a female, the reasons against such a journey may be urged with increased force.

There are, however, chronic cases of consumption, in which the disease of the lungs, even though arrived at its last stage, may derive benefit by a removal to a mild climate. The cases to which I allude, are those in which the disease has been induced in persons little disposed to it constitutionally, and in whom it usually occurs later in life than when hereditary. The tuberculous affection in such persons is occasionally confined to a small portion of the lungs, and the system sympathizes little with the local disease. In instances of this kind, a residence for some time in a mild climate, especially when aided by proper regimen, and such remedies as the state of the general health or any complication requires, may be the means of saving the patient. Likewise, in those fortunate, but unhappily too rare examples of consumption, where the progress of the disease in the lungs has been arrested by nature, but in which a long period must elapse before the work of reparation is completed, a mild climate may be of considerable service in improving the general health, and in removing the patient from many causes which are likely to renew irritation in the lungs. Such a climate, indeed, offers great advantages to consumptive invalids of this description. During my residence abroad, I met with several such who passed their winters in Italy with much more comfort and enjoyment of life than they did in England. I believe that, in nicely balanced cases, life may be preserved for many years by a constant residence in mild climate, and by sedulously avoiding, at the same time, whatever could disturb the balance of the circulation, produce congestion, or light up inflammatory disease in the lungs.

When removal to a mild climate is decided on, the next subject which naturally presents itself for consideration, regards the selection of that which is most suitable to the case. The question has been often put to me—Which is the best climate? The truth is, no one climate or situation is the best in all cases. In the first part of this work I have given the character of the climate of the different places resorted to by invalids, and have endeavoured to draw a comparative view of their respective merits; and to this I beg to refer the reader. With regard to the climates of the south of France and Italy, I may here observe, that for consumptive invalids, in whom there exists much sensibility to harsh and keen winds, and, more especially, if the immediate vicinity of the sea is known to disagree, Rome or Pisa are the best situations for a winter residence. When, on the contrary, the patient labours under a languid or oppressed circulation, with a relaxed habit, and a disposition to congestion or to hæmorrhage rather than to inflammation, and, more especially, where the sea air is known by experience to agree with the individual,—Nice deserves the preference. In cases complicated with gastric irritation, however, Nice is an improper residence, its climate being decidedly inimical to this state. The climate of Hyères may be considered as similar to that of Nice in this respect. The influence of such a morbid condition of stomach in modifying all other diseases, is sufficient to claim for it the chief consideration in deciding upon the particular situation; although, I fear, it is but seldom thought of when the physician is deciding which climate deserves to be preferred. Judging, however, from experience, I should say, that where this state of the stomach exists, a climate which disagrees with it, will do the patient little good, whatever may be the other disease under which he labours.

With those cases of chronic consumption, therefore, to which I have alluded, and which, according to my observation, are almost invariably complicated with, and, I believe, in a large proportion of cases, chiefly induced by disorder of the digestive organs, Nice will decidedly disagree ; and, besides the gastric dyspepsia, such patients have generally an irritated state of the bronchial membrane, with a dry state of the skin and a morbid degree of sensibility of the nervous system,—in all of which states that place is unfavourable. Rome or Pisa will agree better with this class of invalids.

But the climate which of all others I consider the best suited to consumptive patients generally is that of Madeira. It will be seen by a reference to the meteorological tables in the Appendix, and from the comparisons which I have made between the climate of this island and that of the different climates on the continent of Europe in the article on Madeira, that the winter temperature is considerably higher and more equable, and the summer heat much more moderate than at any of these places. To such consumptive patients, therefore, as are likely to derive benefit from climate, I consider Madeira as affording altogether the best residence. And this opinion does not rest merely on a consideration of the physical qualities of this climate, but is warranted by the experience of its effects on those cases of consumption which alone ought to be sent abroad, as will be seen by a reference to Dr. Renton's table.* Madeira has also this advantage (a very great one in my opinion) over all the other places

* See Article on Madeira, p. 150.

in the south of Europe, that the patient may reside there during the whole year, and thus avoid the inconveniences and even risks attending a long journey, to which consumptive invalids who pass the winter in Italy must be exposed. The summer climate of the whole Mediterranean, is unsuited to consumptive invalids, and indeed is known by experience to be so pernicious to them, that sailors and soldiers attacked with the disease in the Mediterranean fleet, and garrisons of Malta, &c., are invariably sent to England on the approach of summer.

But various circumstances require to be taken into consideration in each individual case, before we decide upon a particular climate. The peculiarities and complications of the disease; the patient's ability to bear travelling, or a sea voyage; the means at his command, and the friends by whom he can be attended, are circumstances which must all be taken into consideration, in weighing the comparative merits of different places, and the inconveniences attending all of them, compared with the comforts and quiet of home. These collateral circumstances may render it advisable to recommend the change to one patient, when another, to whose case it is equally applicable, will be better advised to remain in his own country.

There is one circumstance connected with the residence of consumptive patients which has been much talked of, but concerning which the profession is not quite agreed,—I mean the preference to be given to a sea-side or an inland situation. We have indeed no very satisfactory comparisons on this subject, in which the nature of the climate, occupations and habits of life, &c., of the inhabitants have been fairly taken into account, so as to enable us to judge how far the frequency of consumption, in any particular place, may be connected with the nature of the climate, and how much may depend on the mode of living, &c. The question is certainly a very difficult one, and the circumstances connected with it not easily analyzed; hence it is that we have little more than opinions on the subject; and I regret that I have nothing better to offer at present. From all that I have been enabled to learn and observe, consumption is, I think, *cæteris paribus*, more frequent on the sea coast than in the interior; still the greater mildness of many maritime places, as of those on the south-west coast of England, may more than compensate for this difference, especially when these places are resorted to for a part of the year only.

In Italy, Rome is the only place frequented by invalids, sufficiently remote from the sea to be considered as having an inland climate; and here the comparison is certainly in favour of the inland situation. But my impression is, that there is less difference between the sea-side and inland situations, in that range of latitude, than further north; perhaps owing to the greater dryness of the sea-side in southern climates. Of two climates, the physical characters of which being alike favourable, the one on the sea shore and the other inland, I should certainly prefer the latter as a residence for a consumptive patient, either when the disease existed, or was only threatened; but I am ready to admit that this opinion is unsupported by any very accurate or extensive observation.

A sea voyage is another measure, regarding the advantages of which, in consumption, a difference of opinion exists among professional men. My own opinion is, that a voyage is decidedly beneficial in the early stages of consumption, and most of all when the disease is accompanied with hæmoptysis. I believe the unceasing motion of a ship, by the constant exercise which it produces, is a principal agent in this case;* although it seems

---

* This was the opinion of Gregory: " Mea autem sententia, quicquid boni ex navigatione percipitur, ipsi exercitationi præcipue imputandum. . . . . . Ad hunc motum perficiendum, omnium fere corporis musculorum exercitatio modica, crebra, et vix sensibilis requiritur, et hæc exercitatio sine ulla intermissione perficitur ; ita ut quandocumque aliquis navigationem facit, etiamsi in lecto decumbat, vel dormiat, exercitatione vel gestatione saltem utitur. Quicquid igitur boni ab exercitatione æquali, moderata, et continua, in morbo aliquo percipitur, a navigatione, præ omnibus aliis exercitationibus, jure expectandum est."—*De morbis Cæli mutatione medendis.*

also to act in a particular manner on the nervous system. Several striking instances of the beneficial effects of a sea voyage in consumption fell under my notice while in Italy; and Dr. Peebles, of Rome, whose long residence at Leghorn gave him a favourable opportunity of observing the effects of the voyage on consumptive patients sent from England to Pisa, met with many examples of the same kind. On examining the notes of these cases, with which Dr. Peebles favoured me, I found that hæmoptysis had existed in a greater or lesser degree in every one of them ; and this was also the case in the examples which fell under my own observation. The patient being subject to hæmoptysis I should therefore consider as affording an additional reason for recommending a sea voyage.

In the consumptive cases, also, which are complicated with palpitation or increased action of the heart, whether purely functional or depending upon organic disease, I consider a voyage as a useful measure, and much preferable to a land journey. There may exist complications, on the other hand, which would render a voyage unadvisable. When there is much nervous sensibility, a strong disposition to headach, and an irritable state of the stomach, a sea voyage will often disagree. With these exceptions, I should say that a consumptive patient, in whose case a foreign climate is likely to prove useful, had better go by sea than by land, provided a vessel can be obtained with tolerable accommodations. Much depends upon this last circumstance, and much also on the climate or season in which the voyage is made. The motives for preferring a voyage to a journey will be still stronger, when the patient has not the means of travelling in the most comfortable manner. Sailing or cruising for some time would be still preferable to a voyage. For this measure the Atlantic affords a much more favourable climate than the Mediterranean. From the 25th to the 35th degree of latitude, would perhaps be the best climate, although this must be regulated by the season of the year. When a long voyage is objected to, shorter voyages, under favourable circumstances, and repeated at short intervals, might be of essential benefit.

The measures which have been recommended as necessary preparations for a long journey, are equally requisite in the case of a voyage,—much of the benefit of which will depend upon the condition in which the patient is sent to sea, and the regimen he adopts while there. In the advanced periods of consumption, I consider the propriety of a voyage in the same light as I do change of climate ; but of the two modes of conveyance I should prefer a voyage to a land journey.

There is yet another measure in the treatment of consumption which requires some notice in this work, as it has been recommended as a substitute for change of climate. In place of sending consumptive patients to pass the winter in a milder climate, it has been proposed to keep them in rooms artificially heated and maintained at a regulated temperature. With the advocates of such a measure the state of the lungs appears to be the only consideration; but it need not be told, that without improving the general health, which cannot be done without exercise in the open air, all our measures directed to the local disease will be fruitless. We may by such means keep down inflammatory action in these organs, but we shall be favouring the very condition of the system which led to the disease, and the removal of which condition can alone afford the patient a hope of recovery. In the incipient stages of consumption, therefore, I consider such a measure as the most improper that can in general be adopted. In the advanced stages of the disease, on the other hand, when all hopes of recovery have vanished, and when removal to a distant climate is totally useless, life may be prolonged, in many cases, by keeping the invalids in apartments, the temperature of which is regulated in such a manner as to maintain the air in as pure a state as may be. Females will, *cæteris paribus*, bear such a system of confinement better than males, from the circumstance of its being more congenial to their usual habits of life. Also in consumption and chronic bronchial disease occurring in the more advanced periods of life, such a measure promises to be much more frequently beneficial than in early life. In cases of inflammation of the lungs also which have occurred during the winter, confining the patient entirely to the house in a regulated temperature, till all symptoms of the disease have ceased, and until the return of mild weather, will be very judicious, more especially when such a person is hereditarily disposed to consumption. But when a person so circumstanced has the means, he should pass the following winter in a climate where confinement would be unnecessary, and where he might improve his general health by exercise in the open air.

With respect to the length of time which a consumptive invalid may require to pass in a mild climate, in order to overcome the disposition to the disease, no general rule can be given. When it is had recourse to for the removal of the disordered state which precedes tubercular cachexy, a single winter will be of great benefit, or all that may be necessary. When tubercular cachexy is established, and, still more, when there is reason to suspect the presence of tubercles in the lungs, several years may be requisite. When the disease has proceeded still further, I have already expressed my belief that climate, with a few exceptions, will be of little or no service.

T

When, from the influence of climate and other measures, the disease that threatened the lungs has been warded off, or when tubercular disease of these organs has ceased to make progress, the utmost care should be continued to maintain the general health, and to avoid whatever could excite irritation in the lungs; as there will remain a tendency to a return of the constitutional and local disorders, long after the symptoms have disappeared. Where the disease has advanced a step further, and a breach has been made in the lungs by the softening and expectoration of the tuberculous matter, and a cure has still been effected during a residence in a mild climate, the patient should remain there for a considerable time (some years if possible) after every symptom of the disease has disappeared. The same system of treatment and the same air which enabled nature to effect a cure, should be continued, if practicable, till the respiratory organs and constitution generally have accommodated themselves to the new condition of the parts. This may indeed be such that the individual shall not be able to live in any other climate. Wherever he is, such a person must make up his mind to live with great regularity and temperance during the remainder of his life. He will neither bear full living nor much bodily fatigue, though regular and moderate exercise in the open air, and above all riding, will be of the greatest service to him.

Fulness and excitement, especially as affecting the pulmonary organs, are what he has most to fear. Though the disease has ceased to advance, the integrity of the lungs cannot be restored; they must remain diminished in their capacity in proportion to the extent of tuberculous disease which existed in them. The chest can therefore neither be so fully expanded, nor the blood so freely circulated through the lungs as before the disease. Hence, as the capacity of the respiratory organs is diminished relatively to the bulk of the body, there will be a constant tendency to a plethoric state of the pulmonary system; and if the quantity and quality of the food, and degree of bodily exertion, are not adapted to the new condition of the lungs, hæmorrhagy or inflammation of these organs will be the consequence, and may speedily terminate a life, that, by a reasonable degree of attention and prudence, might have been prolonged many years. A mild and moderate diet, with abstinence from every thing exciting, can alone save such persons. The state of the digestive organs requires particular attention, as congestion of the abdominal circulation will speedily lead to a similar state of the pulmonary; and when this plethoric condition of the abdominal and pulmonary circulation exists in a considerable degree, either hæmorrhagy from the bowels, or lungs, or apoplexy, or inflammation of some important organ, cannot fail to be the consequence; and this accordingly is the manner in which many such patients are suddenly carried off.

In conclusion, I would submit the following corollaries as a summary of my views regarding the nature and causes of consumption and its treatment, more especially as connected with the effects of climate.

1*st*, That tubercles in the lungs constitute the essential character and immediate cause of consumption.

2*nd*, That tubercles originate in a morbid condition of the general system.

3*rd*, That such a state of system frequently has for its cause hereditary predisposition; in other instances it is induced by various functional disorders; while in a third class of cases (perhaps the most numerous) it arises from the conjoint effects of both these causes.

4*th*, That consumption is to be prevented only by adopting such means as shall counteract the hereditary predisposition, (where it exists,) and maintain the healthy condition of the various functions from infancy to the full developement of the body.

5*th*, That in the general disorder of the health which leads to tubercular cachexy,—in tubercular cachexy itself, and even when tubercles are formed in the lungs, unattended with much constitutional irritation, a residence in a mild climate will prove beneficial ; and also in cases of chronic consumption, at any stage, when the lungs are not extensively implicated in tubercular disease, and when the system does not sympathize much with the local disorder.

6*th*, That in cases of confirmed consumption, in which the lungs are extensively diseased, and when hectic fever, emaciation, and the other symptoms which characterize its advanced stages are present, change of climate can be of no service, and may even accelerate the progress of the disease.

7*th*, That climate, to be effectual in any case, requires to be continued for a considerable time—in most cases for years.

CHRONIC DISEASES OF THE LARYNX, TRACHEA AND BRONCHIA.

There is no class of complaints in which the beneficial effects of change of air and climate are more speedily manifested, than in irritation of the mucous membranes of the air passages. In the slighter affections of this kind, change of air, to the distance only of a few miles, has often a remarkable effect in removing coughs, sometimes in the course of a few days, which had resisted medical treatment perhaps for weeks. But in protracted cases of this kind, in which the mucous membrane of the bronchia is deeply and extensively affected, the disease assumes a more serious character, and nothing short of a complete change of climate will produce much effect.

This is a step, however, which must not be taken without due deliberation. Every case will not be benefited by the change, nor will the same climate agree with all; and many who would derive benefit from such a measure require some previous treatment. Before the patient leaves his home, we ought to be assured that all acute, and even sub-acute inflammation has ceased, or otherwise such a measure is more likely to increase than to diminish the disease. This is well exemplified in the effects of change of air in common catarrhal affections. A journey in the commencement of a cold generally increases it; if, on the contrary, the acute period of the cold has passed by, a short journey is one of the most effectual means of removing the cough entirely. And the same thing has been long observed in hooping-cough. The acute periods of even the slighter cases of bronchial irritation should, therefore, have passed by before change of air is resorted to as a remedy. Besides the want of any good effect from this measure in the earlier stages of these affections, some of the circumstances necessarily attendant on such a change are in themselves injurious. In no class of cases, perhaps, are rest and quiet more essentially necessary than in the acute and even sub-acute stages of bronchial disease, and it need hardly be stated that these requisites are incompatible with the exigencies of a journey. Were these circumstances respecting the nature and the periods of disease, in which change of air is suitable, more attended to, and the exciting effects of travelling, particularly in hot, dry weather, taken into account, such a change might be made a much more efficient remedy than it ever can be, while it is adopted in the loose and inconsiderate manner in which we too often see it at present. And it is not sufficient in cases of this kind to remove inflammatory action before the journey is commenced; we must point out to our patients the various causes likely to renew it, in order that these may be carefully avoided while travelling. The long continuance of the disease is no reason for the disregard of these precautions, as the most chronic degree of inflammation may be easily excited into a more acute form. It is necessary to impress this fact strongly on the minds of such patients, and of their relations and attendants, as the debility which often accompanies the disease, and is the consequence of it, frequently attracts the principal attention ; and the injudicious measures often adopted to " support the strength," give rise, not unfrequently, to an increase of the disease, or, at least, have the effect of counteracting the beneficial influence of climate.

The next circumstance which requires attention in bronchial diseases, is the state of the digestive organs.   Judging from my own observation, I would say that irritation of the bronchial membrane is very often a sympathetic affection depending upon irritation of the stomach : most assuredly these two pathological states co-exist in a large proportion of cases ; and I think the remark applies in a particular manner to the affections of the larynx and trachea that occur after the middle period of life.   In cases of this kind, upon tracing the progress of the disease, we shall generally find, that the bronchial affection, the " liability to catch cold," the " spring cough," the troublesome " morning phlegm," &c., did not occur till the patient had suffered for some time, often for years, from symptoms of disordered digestive organs. When this is the case, we shall make little progress in the cure of the laryngeal and tracheal diseases, until we have subdued the irritation of the digestive organs; and the hopes of the successful issue of our treatment must therefore rest chiefly on the facility with which this yields to our remedial measures. Indeed, it may be stated generally, that the acute and chronic inflammations of the chest are comparatively of easy management when the digestive organs are in a state of integrity,—when the abdominal circulation is unembarrassed, and the secretions of the various organs connected with digestion, free and natural.* I must therefore repeat the statement made above, that when the stomach and chylopoietic viscera are found on examination to be in an irritated and congested state, our first object should be to restore them to a better condition, before the patient leaves his own country, otherwise the change is far less likely to prove beneficial, and may even be injurious to him.

The state of the skin will also require our particular attention, as it is seldom in a healthy condition in persons that have long laboured under bronchial irritation.

---

* For some very judicious remarks on this subject, I beg to refer to the notes on the article *Pneumonia* in Dr. Forbes' translation of Laennec.

For the management of such invalids during the
journey, I beg to refer to the article on that
subject, and for directions respecting regimen, &c.,
to the article on " Disorders of the Digestive
Organs ;" as these are strictly applicable to the
class of diseases now under consideration. One
remedy, namely warm bathing, which is highly
useful in dyspeptic complaints, requires more
caution in bronchial, and still more in tracheal
and laryngeal irritations, even when complicated
with such complaints. Unless under very convenient circumstances, therefore, the warm bath
had perhaps better be omitted in these cases,
especially during the journey.

Besides these important considerations, which
demand the especial attention of the physician,
and can only be regulated by him, there are some
minor circumstances, still however of consequence,
which claim the notice of the patient more particularly, and respecting which he can often minister
to himself. Some of these I shall now mention.
Persons labouring under irritations of the respiratory organs, should be particularly careful during
the journey (and indeed at all times and in all
climates) to avoid currents of air, cold, damp
places, or long exposure to a chilly, humid atmosphere. Although such persons should take regular
exercise in the open air, when the weather is
favourable, it is far better that they should remain
within doors, than expose themselves to a cold,

moist air or to a cold wind. High wind is particularly injurious to persons labouring under an
irritable state of the bronchial membrane, and
exposure to it, therefore, should be avoided in
every climate; for even when of a mild temperature strong wind proves irritating to such
patients. Remaining long in a cold atmosphere,
(even though this is perfectly calm,) in a state
of inactivity, is also dangerous. The whole surface, and particularly the extremities, become
chilled under such circumstances, and the internal organs congested. A sudden change from
this state to a heated room,—especially if a full
or stimulating meal follows, seldom fails to increase
the bronchial disease; and the same thing is well
known to be a very frequent cause of catarrhal
affections.

To persons suffering from chronic bronchial irritation, or who are very liable to this on exposur
to cold, the application of cold salt and water,
or vinegar and water, to the chest and neck
every morning, followed by diligent friction is
very useful. I know of no measure better calculated than this to give tone to the surface, and
to render it and the subjacent organs less susceptible to the impressions of cold; and, indeed,
the practice of washing the neck and upper part
of the chest with cold water every morning during
the whole year, might be adopted generally with
great advantage in this country, where colds and

inflammatory sore throats are among the most common diseases.* When the weather is fine, and the circumstances in which the patient is placed favourable, the cold sponging may be extended over the whole surface, one part, after it is well rubbed, being thoroughly dried and then covered before another is sponged. The cases in which this practice has appeared to me most useful are languid constitutions, in which there is an unhealthy condition of the mucous system generally. In such subjects, along with a low degree of irritation, there are also a congested state of the mucous membranes, an unhealthy, dry state of the skin, and a relaxed condition of the whole solids, which at once require soothing and bracing.

By means of these ablutions and frictions, or the shower bath and the occasional use of the warm bath, with steady perseverance in a mild regimen and regular exercise, particularly on horseback, a surprising change may often be effected in the health and feelings of such per-

---

* " In my own experience," says Dr. Forbes, " the effect of sponging the chest with cold water and vinegar once or twice a day has proved of immense benefit to delicate subjects, and more especially to those liable to catarrhal affections, and to persons decidedly phthisical. In these cases, although no doubt the practice proves tonic to the system generally, I conceive its chief operation is in lessening the sensibility of the lungs to the impression of cold."—*Translation of Laennec,* 3rd. Edit. p. 98.

sons, and their sensibility to cold greatly diminished. And to this class of invalids one of the greatest advantages of passing a winter in a mild climate is, that these measures, when adopted with judgment, may be continued throughout the whole year.

Warm clothing in all cases of delicate mucous membranes is particularly necessary, and flannel nearest the skin during the day I consider an essential part of this. When the trachea is the part affected, the neck and upper part of the chest should be particularly well covered during the winter and spring with flannel or chamois leather lined with this, or fleecy hosiery; either of which forms an admirable shield against the cold. The lower extremities should be kept especially warm; and I wish it to be understood, that these precautions are as necessary in the south of Europe as in this country; for although, in the former, the weather is altogether considerably warmer and drier, and more steady from day to day, and the winter much shorter than in this country, the alternations of temperature, as I have shown in the first part of this work, are quite as great, while the houses are colder. The spring, too, in the south of Europe, is very irritating, and requires especial caution on the part of the class of invalids for whom I am now writing.

With respect to the best winter residence in

cases of tracheal and bronchial disease, I have no hesitation in giving Rome the general preference : I found it agree more decidedly with my own patients than any other place on the continent ; and I have repeatedly had occasion to compare its influence with that of the other climates upon the same patients. Many of those had previously tried the other places on the continent frequented by invalids, and could thus form a comparison between them. The principal exception which occurs to Rome as the best residence in these cases is, when the disease is accompanied with copious expectoration. In this form of bronchial disease, the climate of Nice generally agrees better. But in the dry tracheal and bronchial affections, accompanied with much irritation, the climate of Rome, and also that of Pisa, is preferable. Independently of any less evident qualities which it may possess, Rome has several obvious advantages over the other residences on the continent, for patients labouring under bronchial irritation. It is little liable to high winds, the air is soft, and the surrounding country is open and well adapted for riding,—the best kind of exercise for this kind of patients.

Even at Rome, however, the invalid labouring under disease of the trachea or bronchia will find reason for much self-denial. He must be cautious in his visits to the cold galleries and churches, and to such of the ancient ruins as

are damp and subject to currents of air, else he
will run the risk of repeated relapses. During a
tramontana storm he should not stir out of doors.
I have known a single ride in one of them produce
a renewal of the disease in a patient who had
been gaining ground several months. These
storms, as I have stated elsewhere, are not frequent, and rarely exceed three days in duration.

In most cases of bronchial disease the climate
of Madeira will, I have no doubt, be more
beneficial than any part of the continent; and
when this affection occurs in young persons disposed to phthisis, I should give it a decided
preference. The best situations in this country
in these affections have been already noticed.*
In the more protracted and obstinate cases of
bronchial disease, a course of mineral water
will often prove of the greatest utility, and very
materially increase the good effects of a residence
in a mild climate. The combined influence of
these two agents will often effect that which
neither alone could. There are several mineral
waters on the continent which have a high reputation, and, I believe deservedly, in this class
of diseases. Of this kind, the springs of EMS on
the Rhine, of BONNES and of CAUTERETS among
the Pyrenees, and of MONT· D'OR in Auvergne, are

* See page 60, &c.

held in the greatest estimation. A residence during one or two winters in Italy at Rome, and a course of one or other of these waters, according to the nature of the case during the summer, afford, I believe, the most effectual means we possess in the more obstinate and deeply rooted cases of this disease.*

The selection of the particular mineral water must depend on the nature of the case. Where the bronchial disease is accompanied with much general delicacy of constitution, and is connected with a congested state of the abdominal circulation, EMS will deserve the preference. In cases of less delicacy, and those especially in which a mountain air promises benefit, or where the

---

* It may appear strange to some of my readers, that so much time should be requisite for the cure of this and some other diseases mentioned in this work, but it must be recollected that I allude to the chronic and more confirmed cases, which, under the usual system of management are never cured, and on which, for the most part, the ordinary resources of our art have been expended before change of climate is adopted. " Medici bene norunt," observes the celebrated Gregory, " multos morbos, quos chronicos vocamus, adeo pertinaces et curatu difficiles esse, ut non nisi longo tempore debellari et sanari possint, etsi optima et efficacissima remedia quotidie adhibeantur : nec ignorant, multa remedia, quæ maxima vi in corpus humanum pollent, per longum tempus usurpare nequire . . . . Novum cælum omnibus aliis remediis longe in hoc præstat, quod non per paucas tantum horas adhiberi potest, sed per plures menses, vel, si opus sit, per annos integros."—*Op. Citat.*

bronchial disease is complicated with chronic cutaneous eruptions, BONNES or CAUTERETS will be more effectual. In cases where there exists a very torpid state of the habit generally, and especially of the skin, or where the occurrence of the bronchial disease has coincided with the disappearance of any cutaneous eruption, the baths of MONT D'OR will, I believe, effect cures where neither of the other waters will. When the mucous membrane of the digestive organs is in a state of chronic irritation at the same time, and when the liver is congested and the bowels torpid, a course of the waters of VICHI may precede those of MONT D'OR with great advantage: and it fortunately happens that the seasons for using the waters at these two places, which are at no great distance from each other, are very convenient for this purpose; June being the best season at the former and July and August at the latter. In some cases, a course of goat's whey, as at Geiss, will be preferable to any of these waters, and may often be combined with the jelly of Iceland moss with great advantage.

It is scarcely necessary, after what has been said on diseases of the mucous membrane of the digestive and respiratory organs, to enter on the subject of similar diseases of the mucous surfaces of other parts. It may suffice to observe, that in chronic irritation of all these membranes, a residence for some time in a mild climate will prove beneficial. In dysmenorrhœa, very generally the consequence of irritation of the mucous membrane of the uterus, and in the other irritations symptomatic of this, among which I may mention the disease of which I have been treating in this article, especially as affecting the larynx, a mild climate will generally prove very beneficial; and great advantage may often be derived, also, from a course of some of the mineral waters mentioned, or, in some cases, from a cold chalybeate water, such as that of Prymont or Spa.

ASTHMA.

Asthma is a term applied, in common language, to various diseases in which difficulty of breathing is a prominent symptom. In technical language it implies a disease in which the difficulty of breathing occurs in paroxysms, after intervals of comparative health. But even when the paroxysm occurs in this manner, and the disease passes for pure asthma, it is still very often by no means a simple spasmodic affection; being very generally complicated with a morbid condition of the bronchia or digestive organs, or of both. Before recommending climate, or any other remedy to an asthmatic patient, therefore, the state of the mucous membranes of the lungs and of the digestive organs, as well as the functions of the different viscera connected with the latter, require to be carefully examined. In almost all the cases of asthma that have fallen under my observation, the digestive organs have been in a state of irritation. The skin of the asthmatic is also very often in a dry, harsh, imperspirable state, and not unfrequently affected with eruptions. And, indeed, so evident is the connection between the state of the skin and this disease in some cases, that the first occurrence of asthma is occasionally dated from the disappearance of some cutaneous complaint, which had been injudiciously removed by local applications, while the cause of it was neglected: this I have known occur at the early age of five years.

In no disease perhaps is the effect of change of climate so conspicuous and so powerful as in asthma. Taking the disease generally, it may be stated that a removal to a warmer climate is highly beneficial; but the degree of relief will depend greatly, more especially in complicated cases, upon the climate being suited to the particular case or complication. We must not, therefore, prescribe for a name, but take into account the pathological condition of the patient, in order that we may be enabled to form an accurate opinion of the disease, and fix upon the climate that is best suited to it.

The following forms of asthma require attention, in prescribing change of air or climate for this disease.

1st, PURE NERVOUS ASTHMA.—It is difficult to say whether Nice, Pisa, or Rome, will agree best with this form of asthma. The general constitution of the patient, and his past experience in the particular quality of air which suits him best, will assist us in deciding. I have not seen a sufficient number of cases of this species abroad to enable me to state any thing very positive on the subject. What passes very often for simple spasmodic asthma will be found, on closer examination, to be complicated with that diseased state of the mucous membrane of the lungs, which has been termed *dry catarrh,*—an affection which generally remains latent for a considerable time, and is very often overlooked; nevertheless it is one of the most frequent causes of asthma. When such a state of the bronchial membrane exists, uncomplicated with gastritic dyspepsia, Nice, I believe, is the best climate for the patient.

2d, SYMPTOMATIC NERVOUS ASTHMA.—The primary irritation in this form is most generally in the stomach, or intestines; sometimes in the uterus. It is also much benefited by a mild climate, but the selection of this must be regulated more from regard to the primary affection, than the secondary one. In most cases of this kind Nice will not agree, and Rome or Pisa will be found better residences.

3d, HUMID ASTHMA.—This is the case in which we have the asthmatic paroxysm occurring at intervals, but with more or less of dyspnœa, cough, and expectoration, at all times. It is asthma complicated with chronic bronchitis, and is one of the most common forms of the disease. This species also may be either idiopathic or symptomatic. The former is commonly much benefited by Nice; the same place is also often useful in the latter variety, but the degree of the benefit will depend on the kind and degree of the gastric affection of which it is symptomatic. On this subject I need not repeat what has been already said in the article on Dyspepsia.

4th, CARDIAC ASTHMA ; or, Asthma complicated with affections of the heart. This form also frequently receives temporary relief from a mild climate. I have known Nice useful in some cases of this kind; but the nature of the primary disease here demands the chief consideration, as upon our power of abating this, must depend mainly our hopes of any permanent effect being produced on the asthma. When change of climate is adopted in this complication, a voyage is much preferable to a land journey.

When asthma is complicated with chronic irritation of the bronchial membrane, or of the digestive organs, or with a congestive state of the hepatic system, or unhealthy state of the skin, a course of warm mineral water will prove of much benefit, by relieving these morbid affections, which often induce and always aggravate asthma.

There is more difficulty in selecting a mineral water for the asthmatic patient than for any other, as the source, most suitable to the other diseases, may be in a situation which decidedly disagrees with the asthma. However well situated the waters of the Pyrenees or of Mont d'Or, might be to the bronchial disease, it would be useless to propose a residence at either of these places, to an asthmatic person who could not breathe at a great elevation, or to send him to Ems or Carlsbad, who could not live in a valley, although the waters of these places might be admirably adapted to the bronchial or abdominal disease. I need not repeat here what I have already stated, regarding the use of mineral waters, under the heads of Dyspepsia and Bronchial diseases, and also when treating of a summer residence for invalids; as the complication of asthma with these disorders is only to be taken into account as far as the air of the place may be suitable for the patient; and on that point we must be chiefly guided by his own past experience.

GOUT.

In the early stages of gout, when the object of the patient is the cure of his disease, and when he possesses the resolution to adhere to such a mode of living as is calculated to remove the gouty disposition entirely, a residence for some time in a mild climate will greatly favour his endeavours.

In the more confirmed cases of this disease, when the joints are permanently affected, and when the general health has suffered, a mild climate very often improves the latter, and prolongs the interval between the paroxysms. The climate of Genoa appears upon the whole most favourable in gout. The disease is more rare there, I believe, than in the other large towns in Italy. I have also known some gouty invalids experience decided benefit from a residence during the winter at Genoa, after they had been disappointed in the effects of the South of France.

The regimen of the gouty invalid residing in the South of Europe, while it requires to be regulated according to the circumstances of the individual case, should also be adapted to the climate. If the disease is in an early stage, and a cure is expected, a very mild regimen is necessary; and as a part of this, a total abstinence from wine is advisable. In the confirmed stages of the disease, the previous habits of the patient must be taken into consideration, in regulating the manner of living. A milder and more moderate diet will, however, be more necessary in Italy than in England. Sweet, acid, white wines should be avoided; but the sound French wines, especially that of Bordeaux, will soon be found to agree with the generality of such invalids; and, contrary to the general belief, prove less "gouty," and less injurious to the health, than the more spirituous wines of Spain, Portugal, and Sicily.

Warm mineral waters, employed both internally and externally, are often beneficial in chronic gout. Having, however, treated minutely of that disease, to which gout is so closely allied, under the head of "Disorders of the Digestive Organs," it is unnecessary to enter into further detail on the present occasion.

CHRONIC RHEUMATISM.

Rheumatism often resists the best directed efforts of medicine; and, after an acute attack, in our own damp, chilly climate, it frequently torments the patient in the chronic form, during the remainder of his life. A residence for some time in a mild climate proves of the greatest benefit in such cases; and is sometimes almost the only measure, which, in the present state of our knowledge, affords a prospect of recovery. Nice and Rome are the places on the continent which, according to my experience, are most beneficial in rheumatism. The preference must be regulated by the peculiarities of the case. Rheumatism is very often complicated with, and frequently kept up by a disordered state of the digestive organs, without the removal of which the affection of the joints can scarcely be cured. In cases of this nature, when gastric irritation of the inflammatory character exists, Rome is the better climate; while, in the pure chronic rheumatism, Nice deserves the preference,—as it does also in those complicated forms of rheumatism, in which the disease exists in combination with an atonic or relaxed state of the stomach. In cachectic rheumatism, or that chronic affection of the joints dependent upon a cachectic state of the system, and when the disease is complicated with anomalous eruptions, Nice and Genoa have appeared to agree particularly well; and Pisa to disagree. Naples and Pau, I consider improper residences in chronic rheumatism, particularly the latter place, where rheumatism is almost endemic.

When a winter passed in Italy fails to remove the rheumatism, I would recommend a course of bathing in some of the mineral waters on the continent, known to be most beneficial in such cases. Aix, in Savoy, has a high character in obstinate affections of this kind, and, I believe, deservedly. The waters of the Pyrenees, as those of CAUTERETS and BAGNÈRES-DE-LUCHON, are also beneficial in similar cases. In Italy, the baths of ISCHIA and of LUCCA, the sulphureous baths of PORRETTA near Bologna, of ABANO near Padua, and, in May, the baths of PISA or of MONTE CATINI in Tuscany, are often used with advantage in rheumatism. When the disease, however, is symptomatic of a

deranged state of the digestive organs, a course
of mineral water, directed with a view to remove
this, will prove more beneficial than any baths
directed only to the affection of the joints; and,
accordingly, I have known a course of the Vichi
waters useful after the baths of the Pyrenees, of
Aix and of Ischia had all failed.

GENERAL DELICACY OF CONSTITUTION IN CHILDHOOD AND YOUTH.

During my residence in the south of Europe,
I found the health of delicate English children,
whether of a strumous habit or otherwise, very
much improved by one or more winters in Italy.
The mildness and dryness of the Italian winter,
and, still more, its shortness, compared to that of
this country, sufficiently explain the beneficial
effects produced on the little invalids. Their delicate frames are not chilled so much nor for so
long a period of the year as in our own climate,
while they are enabled to be much more in the
open air, a circumstance of the greatest importance
to delicate children, and for the want of which
nothing can compensate. I must here, however,
restrict my praise to winter alone, as the summer
in Italy has generally an injurious effect upon such
children, especially if the residence is prolonged
beyond a single season. Under such circumstances

they generally grow rapidly, and become thin, pale, and feeble.*

Rome and Nice are, according to my observation, the best winter residences in such cases. The general characters of their climate, and the opportunities which the surrounding country affords for exercise, give them a superiority over the other towns resorted to by strangers in Italy. The one or other of these places will deserve a preference, according to the form in which the general delicacy or scrofulous disposition shows itself. When there is much gastric irritation, a very frequent occurrence in scrofulous children, Rome will be the more suitable residence. On the other hand, if there is a torpid, languid state of the system generally, and a disposition to relaxation rather than to irritation of the system, Nice will be the preferable climate. When a summer is passed in Italy, Sienna, or the Baths of Lucca, will afford the best residences, or the neighbourhood of Naples, when sea-bathing promises benefit.

There are two periods in early life in scrofulous and delicate constitutions, when a residence for some time in the south of Europe has appeared to me particularly useful. The first is during

---

* The winter in Italy proves useful in difficult dentition, but summer is, in the same degree, pernicious. Infants in Italy should generally be suckled for a longer period than in England; and it is a rule never to wean them in the spring while teething.

childhood, from about the fourth year upwards. At this age children often become delicate and subject to catarrh on slight exposure to cold, to constipated bowels, to swellings of the lymphatic glands, and other symptoms indicating a strumous disposition. This state is occasionally the consequence of the eruptive fevers, as measles or scarlatina. By whatever cause it may have been induced, a residence for some time in a warm climate will prove very beneficial. Even a change to some of the milder situations in our own island, will often prove of great service in such cases. The sea-coast is generally considered the best residence for delicate and scrofulous children and young persons in this country. This, however, is not invariably the case; and even when sea-air may be the best, it is not a matter of indifference what situation is chosen. We have seen that there is a considerable variety of climate among the different places on the sea-coast resorted to by invalids.* For some cases of scrofula, a dry bracing air, such as that of Brighton, will be the most suitable; for others, the more sheltered situation of Hastings; and the milder and softer climate of the south coast of Devon will, in many cases, be a more favourable winter residence than either; while, during the summer months, a dry

---

* See Part the First, p. 20, &c.

elevated part of the interior, such as that afforded by the Malvern Hills, will often be superior to any of these places.

In chronic croup a winter in Italy will also be very useful; for although this disease is generally connected with gastric irritation, it is often induced by exposure to cold and damp, in children predisposed to it. Croup is scarcely known in southern Italy, and no relapses, I believe, occurred during my residence at Rome among English children who had previously had the disease.

When there is a disposition to hydrocephalus, (comparatively a rare disease, I think, in the south of Europe,) and when this is not complicated with much gastric irritation, the same change of climate will be useful.

The diet of the child must, of course, be regulated according to the nature of the case and the climate. Milk does not agree so well in Italy as in England, and should not form so large a proportion of the food of children as it generally and properly does in this country.

The second period of youth at which a mild climate proves decidedly beneficial, is about puberty. It frequently happens at this age, that from pursuing a course of study too assiduously, or from the sedentary habits which are the consequences of it, and from various other causes, the health is materially injured; the system generally becomes debilitated, and the new functions which should take place at this period of life either do not appear, or do so imperfectly, and the general developement of the body is not fully completed. Under such circumstances, a residence for some time in a mild climate becomes a very valuable remedy: when the young person is known to have any hereditary predisposition to consumption the measure is more urgently called for. There exists in such cases a deranged condition of the system which renders it a fit receptacle for the seeds of disease, and which, if not soon corrected, will often terminate in that constitutional disorder which has been termed Tubercular Cachexy, and which we have seen to be the precursor of pulmonary consumption.*

The signs which indicate the state to which I allude are sufficiently evident. The young person loses his usual fulness and strength, the face is generally pale or sallow and the features fallen; the skin pale, often relaxed and moist, more frequently dry and coarse, or this state alternates with general or partial perspirations; cutaneous eruptions are also common; the feet are very liable to become cold, the bowels are constipated, the tongue loaded, and the digestive organs gene-

* See Article on Consumption.

rally disordered. The nervous system is morbidly sensible, the temper is unnaturally irritable, or there is great mental depression, and the whole moral character is often remarkably changed: there is an indifference to the objects and pursuits which previously interested the mind,—there is a degree of languor and disinclination for either bodily or mental exertion; and in females the uterine functions are generally deranged. Scrofula in its more common forms often shows itself, under such circumstances, for the first time.

One of the most powerful means of preventing such consequences when threatened, and of obviating them when they have occurred, is a temporary residence in a warm climate. If this cannot be accomplished the winter should be passed in some of the milder parts of our own island, where by horse exercise, warm sea-bathing, and a well-regulated diet, much may be done to rescue the youthful invalid from the impending danger.

PREMATURE DECAY AT A MORE ADVANCED PERIOD OF LIFE.

About the age of sixty, sometimes much earlier, a remarkable change often takes place in the health without any very obvious cause. The person's appearance becomes greatly changed; his strength is diminished, and he generally becomes thin. He finds himself unequal to the mental and bodily exertions to which he has been long habituated; and the consciousness of this frequently induces a depression of spirits and fretfulness of temper, if these did not already exist as direct effects of the bodily disorder. With the more general evidences of deterioration of health, some organ of importance to life generally shows symptoms of disease. The digestive organs most frequently give indications of suffering, and an habitual morning cough, with more or less of expectoration, often precedes and accompanies this state. Cutaneous eruptions, swellings and pains in the joints, or nervous affections, chiefly of a painful kind, amounting even to tic douloureux, also occasionally occur; or the individual may lapse into a state of general cachexy, without much evident local disease. This, however, is the rarer case, I believe. If such a person is attacked with any acute disease, the constitution often sinks under it with great rapidity.

This state constitutes what is not inaptly termed in common language " a breaking up of the constitution;" which, in truth, it generally proves to be, if not judiciously treated.*

These symptoms of premature decay originate often in too much and long continued mental

---

* See an excellent paper on this disorder under the name of *Climacteric Disease*, by Sir Henry Halford, Bart., President of the Royal College of Physicians.—*Medical Transactions*, Vol. iv., p. 316, &c.

exertion, from close attention to business, and its consequent cares and anxieties; frequently they are the effects of a sedentary life and an habitual system of full living; more frequently still, they are the result of the combined influence of these causes. From whatever cause the above disorder proceeds, a winter passed in Italy, with the adoption of such a regimen, and the use of such other remedial measures as the particular case may require, will prove of essential service in checking its progress, and in restoring the invalid to a state of better health.

When a change of climate cannot be adopted, great benefit may often be obtained from a change of air in our own country, from the use of warm or tepid sea bathing, and a course of such warm mineral waters as are suited to the case.

DISORDERED HEALTH FROM A RESIDENCE IN HOT CLIMATES.

There is still another class of persons to whom a residence of one or more winters in the south of Europe would be of great service in habituating their constitutions to bear a colder climate, before they established themselves finally in this country. I allude to those persons who have resided for a considerable time in a tropical climate, as in the

East or West Indies. By passing the first winter in Italy after their arrival in Europe, their systems will become more gradually habituated to the change in the relative state of the circulation and secretion of the skin and internal organs, which takes place on a removal from a hot to a cold climate. When such persons have suffered from disease of the liver, or from dysentery, this circumstance will afford a still stronger reason for recommending such a measure ; as severe and protracted inflammation of the liver and bowels are rarely completely effaced, and a renewal of these diseases is not an unfrequent consequence of a change from a hot to a cold climate.* Even when there is no formal disease present, the coldness and humidity of the climate of this country during the winter, are fraught with danger to those who have been long resident in the torrid zone. The circulating fluids are thereby forced from the surface and extremities upon the internal organs, and thus disease of the liver and bowels is renewed, or chronic affections of those organs are not unfrequently converted into acute ones : nor is disease of the lungs an unfrequent occurrence

---

* For some very judicious advice to persons returning from a warm climate to this country, the reader is referred to Dr. James Johnson's comprehensive and valuable work on *The Influence of Tropical Climates on European Constitutions, &c.* p. 556, et seq. 4th. Ed.

in such cases.* The great object with individuals so circumstanced, should be to maintain the temperature of the surface and extremities, and an

---

* The great prevalence of pulmonary diseases among the natives of tropical climates who come to this and other cold countries, is doubtless chiefly owing to the influence of a cold and humid atmosphere upon their system. It is in such persons, and in young children, that tuberculous diseases are most speedily induced, and it is in these that inflammation appears more intimately connected with the production of tubercles. The rapid progress of the disease in both classes of persons is to be explained, principally, I believe, by the circumstance of their habit of body being that which is most disposed to tuberculous affections,— the most nearly allied to the tuberculous diathesis. The same disposition to tuberculous diseases is observed in animals brought from warm climates. The monkies that die in the Jardin des Plantes at Paris are, I believe, generally found to be tuberculous; in this case, however, other causes besides cold contribute to induce the same state. The influence of climate on the natives of different countries is often observed on a large scale on white and black troops. According as the former move southward pulmonary diseases become more rare, and the mortality is chiefly from fevers and bowel complaints : as the latter move northwards, or are in any way exposed to cold, pulmonary diseases, frequently of a tuberculous character, become very frequent; much more so than among the European troops. For some interesting facts on this subject, I beg to refer to an excellent paper, by Professor Alison "On the Pathology of Scrofulous Diseases" in the Transactions of the Medico Chirurgical Society of Edinburgh, vol. I., to Mr. Annesley's work on the "Diseases of India," to Mr. Marshall's "Medical Topography of Ceylon," &c., and to a sensible paper by my respected friend, Dr. Whitlaw Ainslie, "On the Constitutions Best Suited to the Climate of India."—*Asiatic Journal*, Vol. XXV.

active state of the cutaneous circulation and secretions : warm clothing, regular and daily exercise, friction by means of a flesh brush, and the habitual and frequent use of the warm bath are, after a mild climate, the most effectual measures for this purpose.

When the biliary system is greatly deranged, a frequent occurrence with natives of this country who have passed some time in India, a course of warm mineral waters, such as those of Carlsbad, of Ems, or of Vichi, &c., will prove very useful, particularly after a winter spent in the south of Europe. These waters are frequently found to remove the biliary symptoms, indigestion, low spirits, &c., by restoring a regular and healthy action of the liver, of the bowels and of the skin.

NAMES OF THE PLACES.	Mean Annual Temp.	Winter	Spring	Sumr.	Autmn.	Jan.	Feb.	March	April	May	June	July	Aug.	Sept.	Oct.	Nov.	Dec.
LONDON, 1. (A.)	50.59	39.12	48.76	62.32	51.35	37.36	40.44	42.64	48.00	55.64	60.00	63.43	63.52	58.80	51.78	43.47	39.58
Edinburgh, 2. (A.)	47.31	39.40	44.70	57.30	47.86	40.17	39.54	39.60	45.84	48.67	54.85	59.31	57.74	55.61	48.37	39.60	38.50
Leith, 3. (A.)	48.36	40.59	45.75	58.27	48.90	41.09	40.62	40.86	46.37	48.01	56.09	60.36	58.37	56.31	49.22	41.19	39.77
Kinfauns, 4.	47.02	39.82	44.60	56.82	46.90	41.25	39.85	38.65	45.17	49.96	55.61	58.39	56.48	53.43	46.38	40.58	38.35
Dublin, 5. (D.)	49.10	39.20	47.30	59.54	50.00	35.42						61.16					
County of Antrim, 6.	47.87	36.75	46.75	58.16	49.83	32.00	38.75	41.25	49.75	49.25	53.75	60.75	60.00	54.25	51.50	43.75	49.50
Kendal, 7.	46.22	36.16	43.79	57.33	46.53	34.88	38.50	38.19	43.21	50.99	55.80	58.10	58.21	52.70	46.29	40.59	35.10
Alderley, (Cheshire,) 8. (A.)	46.80	37.58	45.80	57.10	48.26	36.75	38.50	41.00	45.10	51.30	56.45	57.75	57.20	54.30	48.10	42.40	37.50
New Malton, (Yorkshire,) 9.	47.55	37.79	44.94	59.44	48.65	36.25	38.44	38.51	45.13	51.08	56.40	62.43	59.60	56.06	47.40	42.48	38.70
Oxford, 10.	48.64	37.00	47.10	60.30	50.00	36.90	37.10	42.10	46.70	52.70	58.70	61.60	60.80	57.10	49.40	43.60	37.00
Environs of London. 11. (A.)	48.81	37.20	48.06	60.90	49.13	34.16	41.51	41.51	47.60	53.50	59.15	64.30	61.35	56.22	50.94	44.10	37.66
Bushey Heath, 12.	49.82	38.62	47.06	61.48	51.46	37.95	38.60	40.10	47.60	53.66	59.15	64.20	61.10	59.60	50.70	44.10	35.30
Chichester, 12. (A.)	49.50	38.85	47.75	60.78	51.62	37.95	38.60	39.58	49.29	52.78	59.12	63.00	61.02	58.67	50.54	42.72	39.24
Gosport, 14.	50.24	40.44	47.63	62.00	50.88	40.44	40.94	42.94	47.00	53.00	61.00	63.00	62.00	58.00	50.99	44.45	38.94
Isle of Wight, 15.	51.00	40.31	49.00	63.09	51.63	38.35	40.56	44.75	49.29	59.00	62.00	63.00	62.38	58.00	51.90	44.76	40.60
Cheltenham, 16.	51.32	40.60	50.28	64.33	50.96	38.25	41.75	46.18	50.50	54.16	61.50	66.33	65.12	59.06	50.32	43.50	41.75
Sidmouth, 17.	52.10	40.43	50.66	63.83	53.50	38.30	42.00	45.00	51.00	56.00	61.00	65.00	65.00	61.00	53.00	48.00	43.00
Helston, (Cornwall,) 18.	50.94	43.16	48.76	59.16	52.67	38.40	43.22	44.64	47.23	54.42	59.68	59.68	60.66	56.64	53.19	48.18	46.81
Penzance, 19. (A.)	52.16	44.66	49.66	60.50	53.83	43.00	44.50	46.50	48.50	54.00	59.00	61.00	61.50	58.00	54.50	49.00	46.50
Geneva, 20. (A.)	49.89	33.83	48.90	64.99	50.97	32.00	35.50	41.50	47.30	58.00	62.70	65.50	66.70	59.70	50.70	42.50	34.00
Paris, 21. (A.)	51.50	38.43	48.90	64.47	52.30	35.60	40.50	43.50	49.60	58.10	62.50	65.70	65.50	60.40	52.40	44.20	39.20
Nantes, 22.	55.62	42.23	53.10	70.73	56.41	40.86	43.37	44.37	52.42	60.57	69.62	73.80	69.85	65.85	55.25	50.31	45.60
Bourdeaux, 23.	56.48	42.08	56.46	70.88	56.30	41.00	44.96	46.80	55.79	62.31	73.04	73.04	68.19	65.80	54.34	46.79	41.53
Pau, 24.	54.95	41.79	54.96	67.41	55.64	38.89	44.96	46.50	55.79	62.31	62.31	71.73	68.19	65.80	54.34	46.79	41.53
Montpelier, 25.	57.60	44.20	53.33	71.30	61.30	42.00	45.00	47.00	53.00	60.00	67.00	72.00	75.00	71.00	61.00	52.00	46.00
Avignon, 26. (A.)	58.20	42.60	57.13	74.66	53.00	42.00	43.50	50.50	55.00	66.00	72.00	76.00	76.00	67.00	60.00	50.00	43.30
Marseilles, 27. (A.)	59.50	46.50	57.56	72.50	60.08	45.06	45.06	49.07	55.50	68.00	70.00	76.00	79.00	64.00	58.20	50.40	46.60
Toulon, 28.	59.90	43.30	53.70	74.30	59.00	40.00	44.00	48.00	55.00	68.00	70.00	74.00	79.00	64.00	62.00	51.00	46.00
Nice, 29. (A.)	59.48	47.82	56.23	72.96	61.63	45.85	49.00	51.45	57.00	63.00	69.00	73.50	74.30	69.35	61.85	53.70	48.60
Genoa, 30.	60.37	44.57	56.40	75.03	62.94	41.65	47.47	51.07	57.00	64.45	73.50	75.10	76.50	73.90	64.70	51.05	45.60
Baths of Lucca, 31.	55.00																
Camajore, (Lucca,) 32. (A.)	58.02	44.10	56.32	71.66	59.58	43.60	45.00	50.00	53.70	63.25	68.25	73.00	72.75	67.75	59.50	51.50	45.50
Sienna, 33.	55.60	40.50	54.10	70.80	57.10	39.70	40.22	46.20	53.70	62.40	68.25	72.80	72.30	66.00	58.30	47.10	41.70
Florence, 34.	59.00	44.30	56.00	74.00	60.70	41.00	45.00	48.00	56.00	64.00	69.00	77.00	76.00	70.00	59.00	53.00	47.60
Leghorn, 35. (A.)	59.00	46.30	57.60	74.10	62.00	43.50	45.90	51.70	56.80	64.30	70.60	75.80	74.80	73.50	58.20	53.20	47.70
Pisa, 36.	60.60	46.30	57.20	75.15	62.80	44.00	48.11	51.52	56.30	63.75	70.50	77.50	77.50	69.50	62.62	52.30	47.00
Rome, 37. (A.)	60.70	48.99	57.65	72.16	63.96	47.65	49.45	52.00	56.40	63.75	69.17	73.30	74.02	69.50	63.60	58.80	49.62
Naples, 38. (A.)	61.40	48.50	58.50	70.83	64.50	46.50	48.50	52.00	57.00	66.50	71.00	75.00	76.60	72.50	65.00	54.50	50.50
Mediterranean, gea. temp. of 38. (s.)	67.11	57.63	65.50	76.25	69.10	57.23	57.60	62.64	63.88	70.00	72.08	76.63	80.05	75.28	69.71	62.31	58.05
Cadiz, 39.	62.88	52.90	59.53	70.43	65.35	51.40	53.73	55.21	59.64	63.75	68.16	70.27	72.86	70.17	67.10	58.80	53.58
St. Michaels, (Azores,) 39. (C.)	62.40	57.83	61.17	68.33	62.33	59.00	59.00	59.50	61.00	63.00	67.00	68.00	70.00	68.00	63.00	56.00	55.60
Madeira, 40. (A.)	64.66	62.90	62.90	69.33	67.23	59.00	58.50	59.60	62.50	63.00	65.00	70.00	71.50	71.50	67.50	69.70	60.50
Santa Cruz, (Canary Isles) 41.	70.94	64.65	68.87	76.68	74.17	63.84	64.99	67.17	67.32	72.12	73.89	77.27	78.89	77.43	74.66	70.43	65.82
Cairo, 42.	72.17	58.52	73.58	85.10	71.48	58.10	56.12	64.58	77.90	78.26	83.66	85.82	85.82	79.16	72.32	69.96	61.34

TABLE II.—SHOWING THE DIFFERENCE BETWEEN THE MEAN TEMPERATURE OF EACH SEASON AND BETWEEN THE MEAN TEMPERATURE OF EACH MONTH.

NAMES OF THE PLACES.	Annual Mean Temperature.	Difference of the Mean Temperature of Winter and Summer.	Difference of the Mean Temperature of warmest and coldest months.	Mean Difference of Successive Months.	DIFFERENCE OF THE SUCCESSIVE SEASONS.				DIFFERENCE OF THE SUCCESSIVE MONTHS.											
					of Winter and Spring	of Spring and Summer	of Summer and Autumn	of Autumn and Winter	of January and Feb.	of Feb. and March	of March and April	of April and May	of May and June	of June and July	of July and August	of August and Sept.	of Sept. and October	of October and Nov.	of Nov. and Dec.	of Dec. and January
LONDON	50.39	23.20	26.17	4.36	9.64	13.56	11.00	12.22	3.08	2.20	5.36	7.64	4.36	3.43	0.10	4.73	7.00	8.31	3.89	2.22
Environs of London	48.81	23.60	28.24	4.87	10.86	12.74	11.67	11.93	5.62	1.73	5.88	9.90	2.87	3.74	1.05	5.13	6.00	9.31	3.27	3.50
Edinburgh . . .	47.31	17.90	20.81	3.65	5.30	12.60	9.44	8.46	0.63	0.06	6.24	3.17	6.18	4.48	1.57	2.13	7.24	8.77	1.10	1.67
Leith	48.36	17.68	20.59	3.52	5.16	12.52	9.37	8.31	0.47	0.24	5.51	3.64	6.08	4.27	1.99	2.06	7.11	8.03	1.42	1.32
England generally	49.51	21.69	24.54	4.38	8.50	12.91	10.71	11.33	3.04	2.18	4.31	9.18	5.23	2.84	1.00	4.07	6.70	6.75	4.65	2.70
Scotland . . .	46.36	18.88	21.72	3.52	6.36	12.46	10.03	8.81	0.46	0.45	5.53	4.86	5.86	3.36	1.93	3.14	6.36	7.01	2.59	1.65
County of Antrim	47.87	21.39	28.75	4.87	10.09	11.41	8.33	13.08	6.75	2.50	8.50	0.50	4.50	7.00	0.75	5.75	2.70	7.75	4.25	7.50
Kendal	46.22	21.17	23.33	3.94	7.63	13.54	10.80	10.37	3.62	0.31	5.02	7.78	4.81	2.30	0.11	5.51	6.41	5.70	5.49	0.22
Geneva	49.69	31.16	34.56	5.76	15.7	16.09	14.02	17.14	3.50	0.00	5.70	10.80	4.70	3.86	0.86	6.00	9.00	8.20	8.50	2.00
Paris	51.00	25.83	29.50	4.91	12.00	13.90	11.00	14.83	4.50	2.80	5.20	10.00	3.00	4.00	0.50	5.00	7.00	7.00	8.00	2.00
Penzance . . .	52.16	15.84	18.50	3.05	5.00	10.84	6.67	9.17	1.50	2.00	2.00	5.50	5.00	2.00	0.50	3.50	3.10	5.50	2.50	3.50
South-West of France	55.99	26.42	30.87	4.47	12.08	14.59	12.74	14.00	4.55	1.45	8.52	7.33	4.52	6.80	3.72	3.22	11.08	6.27	5.27	3.94
South-East of France	58.82	29.26	35.33	5.66	11.66	17.75	13.36	16.7	2.19	4.25	5.83	10.33	5.00	4.33	2.66	9.33	6.33	8.96	6.37	3.40
Nice	59.48	23.57	28.22	4.70	9.50	14.52	10.01	13.00	3.07	2.72	4.20	7.40	5.00	4.25	2.00	4.00	9.50	7.00	5.05	2.90
Italy	59.46	27.56	32.10	5.75	11.53	16.03	11.33	16.70	3.50	4.33	6.21	7.63	5.80	5.12	0.82	4.30	9.53	9.06	5.85	3.40
Madeira , . .	64.56	9.83	14.50	2.41	2.70	7.13	2.10	7.23	1.00	2.56	1.44	0.50	2.00	5.00	3.00	1.50	4.00	4.80	2.20	1.00
Santa Cruz . .	70.94	12.03	15.05	2.51	4.22	7.81	2.51	9.52	0.45	2.88	0.15	4.80	1.77	3.38	1.62	1.46	2.77	4.23	4.61	2.00
Cairo	72.17	26.58	27.72	5.30	15.06	11.58	13.62	13.00	2.00	8.46	13.32	0.36	5.40	2.16	0.00	6.66	6.84	10.64	1.61	3.24

TABLE III.—CONTAINING THE ANNUAL AND MONTHLY RANGES OF TEMPERATURE.

NAMES OF THE PLACES.	Mean Annual Temperature.	Annual Range. Range	Maximum of the Year	Minimum of the Year	Mean of the Monthly Ranges	January. Range	Maximum	Minimum	February. Range	Maximum	Minimum	March. Range	Maximum	Minimum	April. Range	Maximum	Minimum	May. Range	Maximum	Minimum	June. Range	Maximum	Minimum	July. Range	Maximum	Minimum	August. Range	Maximum	Minimum	September. Range	Maximum	Minimum	October. Range	Maximum	Minimum	November. Range	Maximum	Minimum	December. Range	Maximum	Minimum
London, 1. (B.)	50.39	*64	86	22	*34	28	50	22	27	52	25	32	61	29	37	69	32	39	75	36	48	86	38	33	77	44	38	82	44	35	75	40	33	65	32	30	57	27	30	54	24
Alderley, 8. (B.)	46.80	*58	76	18	*34	32	50	18	30	52	22	35	58	23	39	66	27	39	71	32	37	76	39	31	74	43	32	74	42	37	73	36	30	62	32	31	56	25	32	51	19
Environs of London, 11. (B.)	48.81	*67	83	16	*38	33	49	16	35	54	19	36	60	24	43	69	26	45	78	33	41	80	39	42	83	41	37	79	42	41	75	34	38	68	30	34	56	22	33	53	20
Gosport, 14	50.24	*66	80	14	*31	34	54	20	42	56	14	28	60	32	35	70	35	32	72	40	30	75	45	27	80	53	29	77	48	24	73	49	33	68	35	35	62	27	26	57	31
Cheltenham, 16.	51.32	*60	85	25	*31	25	50	25	23	53	30	33	61	28	36	68	32	35	71	36	36	79	43	38	85	47	33	81	48	31	74	43	30	65	35	28	57	29	27	55	28
Sidmouth, 17.	52.10	*53	74	21	*30	26	47	21	25	52	27	30	56	26	29	60	31	28	66	38	32	73	41	32	74	42	32	74	42	32	71	39	33	64	31	30	57	27	29	54	25
Penzance, 19. (B.)	52.16	*49	76	27	*24	26	54	28	22	55	33	25	59	34	26	62	36	27	68	41	26	72	46	22	73	51	22	73	51	23	69	46	24	64	40	21	57	36	22	56	34
Pau, 24.	54.95	68	89	21	28	35	56	21	25	60	35	30	65	35	28	71	43	29	80	51	28	80	52	30	89	59	24	82	58	30	82	52	24	70	46	25	64	39	31	56	25
Montpelier, 25.	57.60	59	86	27	23	26	53	27	27	55	28	23	58	35	23	64	41	22	71	49	24	80	56	23	85	62	21	86	65	20	75	55	23	71	48	22	62	40	25	57	32
Nice, 29.	59.48	60	87	27	21	31	58	27	21	58	37	24	65	41	23	69	46	26	77	41	20	78	58	15	81	66	18	87	69	21	82	61	22	70	48	18	61	43	19	59	40
Rome, 37.	60.70	62	91	29	28	29	58	29	29	60	31	28	65	37	30	74	44	28	80	52	28	88	60	27	91	64	29	91	62	30	85	55	31	77	46	28	67	39	29	60	31
Naples, 38.	61.40	64	93	29	29_	29	58	29	29	60	31	31	69	38	35	78	43	35	86	51	32	88	56	29	93	64	29	91	62	28	88	60	28	79	51	20	64	44	27	61	34
Madeira, 40. (B.)†	68.89	23	77	54	12	12	68	56	11	68	57	13	67	54	13	71	58	15	75	60	14	76	62	12	77	65	10	77	67	11	77	66	11	76	65	12	71	59	11	69	50
Idem, (°)	64.56	*35	85	50	*18	19	69	50	17	68	51	18	69	51	17	72	55	20	75	55	15	73	58	13	76	63	17	82	65	21	85	64	19	77	58	20	72	52	16	68	52

* The observations made in England, as denoted by the asterisk, were made with the register thermometer, and, consequently, give a much greater range there than abroad, where, with the exception of Madeira, the observations are confined to the day.

TABLE IV.—CONTAINING THE DAILY RANGE OF TEMPERATURE.

NAMES OF THE PLACES.	Annual Mean Temperature.	Range of daily Temperature for the Year.		January.		February.		March.		April.		May.		June.		July.		August.		September.		October.		November.		December.	
		Mean daily Range	Extreme daily Range	Mean daily Range	Extreme daily Range	Mean daily Range	Extreme daily Range	Mean daily Range	Extreme daily Range	Mean daily Range	Extreme daily Range	Mean daily Range	Extreme daily Range	Mean daily Range	Extreme daily Range	Mean daily Range	Extreme daily Range	Mean daily Range	Extreme daily Range	Mean daily Range	Extreme daily Range	Mean daily Range	Extreme daily Range	Mean daily Range	Extreme daily Range	Mean daily Range	Extreme daily Range
London, 1. (c.)	50.39	*11	:	7	:	9	:	11	:	13	:	16	:	18	:	16	:	7	:	13	:	11	:	8	:	7	:
Leith, 3. (B.)	48.36	6	:	3	:	4	:	6	:	10	:	8	:	8	:	10	:	8	:	8	:	5	:	4	:	2	:
Alderley, 8. (c.)	46.80	6.6	:	5	:	6	:	8	:	9	:	8	:	7	:	6	:	6	:	8	:	6	:	6	:	4	:
Environs of London, 11. (c.)	48.81	*15	:	9	:	12	:	14	:	19	:	19	:	20	:	19	:	18	:	18	:	15	:	11	:	10	:
Chiswick, 13.	....	*15	:	9	:	7	:	12	:	17	:	18	:	17	:	23	:	24	:	18	:	16	:	12	:	9	:
Idem,	....	9	:	5	:	6	:	10	:	11	:	11	:	12	:	11	:	11	:	10	:	9	:	6	:	5	:
Gosport, 14.	50.24	6.1	*25	6	18	7	21	6	24	7	22	5	21	6	24	7	25	7	23	7	24	5	21	5	19	5	17
Sidmouth, 17.	52.10	...	16	...	13	...	12	...	12	...	13	...	11	...	16	...	10	...	9	...	11	...	15	...	11	...	13
Penzance, 19. (c.)	52.16	6.7	:	4	:	6	:	8	:	9	:	9	:	8	:	8	:	8	:	7	:	6	:	5	:	3	:
Geneva, 20. (B.)	49.89	12.5	:	7	:	10	:	13	:	15	:	16	:	16	:	16	:	17	:	14	:	11	:	8	:	7	:
Nantes, 22.	55.62	5.7	:	3	:	4	:	5	:	8	:	3	:	6	:	10	:	7	:	9	:	6	:	4	:	4	:
Pau, 24. (B.)	54.95	7.6	20	7	16	9	16	9	17	8	18	10	16	8	15	8	20	5	14	7	14	5	14	4	15	4	13
Montpelier, 25.	57.60	12.0	:	8	:	9	:	14	:	14	:	14	:	15	:	15	:	17	:	13	:	19	:	10	:	7	:
Avignon, 26. (B.)	58.20	12.5	:	8	:	8	:	10	:	12	:	15	:	19	:	19	:	17	:	15	:	12	:	8	:	7	:
Nice, 29. (B.)	59.60	8.5	18	7	16	9	18	9	17	11	18	10	16	8	14	10	15	11	12	8	16	7	16	6	17	6	14
Camajore, 32.	58.07	10.8	:	7	:	9	:	10	:	11	:	12	:	14	:	14	:	13	:	12	:	11	:	7	:	6	:
Sienna, 33.	55.60	15.0	:	11	:	14	:	16	:	21	:	21	:	17	:	17	:	17	:	16	:	14	:	11	:	10	:
Rome, 37. (B.)	60.70	11.0	20	11	16	10	18	12	19	10	20	10	17	9	16	11	16	13	18	12	17	14	20	10	17	9	13
Naples, 38. (B.)	61.40	13.3	23	9	14	11	19	11	18	14	20	17	21	16	22	16	23	17	21	15	21	14	18	11	14	9	15
Madeira, 40. (c.)	64.56	*10.0	17	11	17	9	13	10	14	9	13	8	11	8	10	10	12	12	15	16	17	16	16	10	15	11	14

* The asterisk indicates where the observations were made by a register thermometer, and thus give the range of the whole twenty-fours, whilst the others give the range of the day only.

TABLE V.—SHOWING THE VARIATIONS OF TEMPERATURE BETWEEN EACH SUCCESSIVE DAY, FOR EACH MONTH AND FOR THE WHOLE YEAR.

NAMES OF THE PLACES	Mean annual Temp.	Mean Var. of successive days	Mean of Extreme Var. Rise	Fall	Absolute Extreme Var. Rise	Fall	Jan Mean Var	Jan Gr. Rise	Jan Gr. Fall	Feb Mean Var	Feb Gr. Rise	Feb Gr. Fall	Mar Mean Var	Mar Gr. Rise	Mar Gr. Fall	Apr Mean Var	Apr Gr. Rise	Apr Gr. Fall	May Mean Var	May Gr. Rise	May Gr. Fall	Jun Mean Var	Jun Gr. Rise	Jun Gr. Fall	Jul Mean Var	Jul Gr. Rise	Jul Gr. Fall	Aug Mean Var	Aug Gr. Rise	Aug Gr. Fall	Sep Mean Var	Sep Gr. Rise	Sep Gr. Fall	Oct Mean Var	Oct Gr. Rise	Oct Gr. Fall	Nov Mean Var	Nov Gr. Rise	Nov Gr. Fall	Dec Mean Var	Dec Gr. Rise	Dec Gr. Fall
LONDON, 1.(D)	50.39	4.01	14.33	14.85	18.00	21.00	5.10	16.00	15.00	3.20	12.00	8.00	3.35	15.0	12.0	4.60	12.0	21.0	3.8.	17.0	13.0	4.60	15.0	20.6	3.50	12.0	12.0	3.20	15.0	14.0	3.50	11.0	17.0	4.30	12.0	15.0	4.70	18.0	17.0	4.80	17.0	14.0
CHISWICK, (nr. London,) (13)		4.03	16.00	14.40	22.0	18.00	3.80	14.00	12.0	4.20	16.00	16.00	4.00	18.0	16.0	4.40	18.0	14.0	3.71	14.0	13.0	3.8.	13.0	12.0	3.70	14.0	14.0	3.40	13.0	12.0	4.3.	16.0	14.0	4.9.	22.0	18.0	4.20	17..	17.0	4.00	16.0	15.0
PENZANCE, 19. (D.)	52.00	2.68	8.64		10.00		3.74	10.56		3.26	10.0.		3.15	10.5		2.52	8.00		2.0.	5.60		1.61	5.56		1.46	5.00		1.27	4.6.		2.55	9.2.		3.02	9.0.		2.1.	11.2.		4.41	12,50	
PARIS, 21. (C.)	51.50	3.90					4.10			3.75			4.2.			4.00			3.7.			4.60			3.26			3.40			3.75			3.7.			4.40			3.75		
PAU, 24. (C.)	54.95	3.55	8.9.	9.90	10.50	13.50	3.84	10.3.	10.00	4.16	10.50	9.85	3.42	9.83	11.16	4.24	9.85	11.66	4.00	7.5.	13.50	3.76	10.30	8.8.	4.23	10.1.	12.86	3.2.	7.80	10.36	2.91	7.66	13.0.	2.7	6.84	10.56	2.47	6.8.	8.66	3.67	9.33	11.1.
NICE, 29. (C.)	59.48	2.33	6.2.	7.2.	11.2.	12.2.	2.60	8.20	6.40	3.00	11.20	12.2.	2.40	8.00	8.0.	4.00	6.4.	8.60	2.2.	4.60	6.4.	2.26	5.0.	7.2.	1.5.	3.5.	4.5.	1.5.	4.30	4.6.	1.75	6.20	6.80	2.6.	5.2.	7.75	1.9.	5.0.	7.50	2.40	5.00	6.44
FLORENCE, 34.	59.00	2.90	7.60	8.01	10.00	11.00	3.3.	10.00	9.25	2.6.	7.-0	7.00	3.00	9.12	7.5.	2.8.	8.09	8.00	3.00	8.00	10.6.	2.6.	9.2	5.5	3.00	7.00	11.0	2.15	4.00	7.0.	2.2.	5.80	8.05	3.5.	7.7.	8.09	3.75	6.60	8.00	2.80	8.85	6.2.
LEGHORN, 35.	60.00	2.44	6.10	7.7.	12.0.	1.8	3.1	12.00	2.8.	2.41	6.60	8.4.	2.16	8.40	7.10	3.33	8.95	8.90	6..	6..	5.3.	1.3.	3.70	3.3	2.5.	10.0.	8.00	1.50	4.0.	4.00	2.67	8.00	10.00	2.8.	10.0.	10.00	3.50	6.60	8.00	2.45	8.90	7.2.
ROME, 37. (C.)	60.70	2.80	6.2.	8.5.	13.50	15.30	3.0.	9.50	8.40	3.0.	5.60	8.20	2.8.	7.50	8.20	2.82	8.40	9.00	2.80	7.8.	7.20	2.6.	80	8.5.	2.4.	6.5.	9.5.	2.06	8.60	8.60	2.56	6.46	6.66	3.00	8.00	9.2.	3.50	8.80	11.60	3.45	10.50	9.2.
NAPLES, 1b. (C.)	61.40	3..6	7.0.	8.54	10.75	13.86	2.80	7.50	8.00	2.86	6.60	10.75	4.06	6.6.	4.06	2.90	7.8.	9.50	4.00	8.3.	8.3.	7.66	8.8.	8.8.	3.09	6.40	8.64	2.40	8.64	8.64	2.46	6.00	8.40	4.00	5.80	8.20	1.90	4.60	9.50	3.00	8.20	8.66
CADIZ, 39. (B.)	62.88	1.00					1.2.			1.25			0.7			1.23			1.00			0.75			0.5.			1.50			1.25			1.50			1.00			1.00		
MADEIRA,40.(D)	64.56	1.11	5.00	5.41	8.01	8.0.	1.8.	6.00	6.00	1.40	8.00	5.00	0.90	4.00	6.00	1.33	5.00	8.00	0.90	4.00	5.00	0.80	4.00	3.00	0.70	0.2.	0.30	0.80	3.00	5.00	1.23	4.00	5.00	1.13	3.00	5.00	1.10	6.60	6.00	1.23	4.00	6.00

TABLE VI.—SHOWING THE MEAN TEMPERATURE OF THE SAME HOURS OF THE DAY AT DIFFERENT PLACES.

The spanning headers are: "Mean Temperature of the Seasons at each particular hour" covers Winter / Spring / Summr. / Autmn.; "Mean Temperature of the months at each particular hour" covers Jan.–Dec.

Hours of the day	Names of the Places	Years of Observation	Mean Temperature of the Year	Mean Temperature of the Year for particular Hours	Mean Annual Temperature of each particular hour more or less than mean annual Temperature of 24 hrs.	Winter	Spring	Summr.	Autmn.	Jan.	Feb.	Mar.	April	May	June	July	Aug.	Sept.	Oct.	Nov.	Dec.	Names of Observers
A.M. Sun Rise	LONDON	10 years	50.°89	44.°00	−6.°59	35.°80	42.°02	54.°90	46.°02	35.°4	35.°3	37.°3	41.°8	47.°4	52.°2	55.°7	56.°6	52.°4	46.°2	40.°1	36.°7	Howard, *Lower mean.*
	Environs of London	1824—1825	48.81	41.10	−7.71	31.90	39.47	51.30	41.60	29.3	33.7	34.5	37.7	46.0	52.9	55.0	54.6	52.4	42.7	35.0	32.7	Idem, *Lower mean.*
	Leith	1803—1812	48.36	45.20	−3.16	39.30	41.30	53.20	46.80	40.1	39.2	37.9	40.5	45.4	51.8	53.3	54.6	52.8	47.5	40.0	39.1	Brewster, *Leith Fort Observations.*
	Geneva	1802—1806	49.89	44.60	−5.29	29.83	41.50	56.93	45.66	38.5	39.2	37.9	39.5	50.0	51.8	58.0	58.0	53.0	48.0	38.5	30.5	Pictet, *Bibliotheque Universelle.*
	Avignon	1777—1816	58.07	52.36	−5.84	39.90	50.66	65.93	53.66	38.3	38.4	43.5	50.5	57.7	63.9	65.9	68.0	61.0	53.5	46.5	41.3	M. Guérin, *Musée Culvet.*
	Camajore, (Lucca)	1823—1826	58.07	52.40	−5.57	40.90	50.00	64.80	51.00	40.2	40.5	45.0	50.5	57.5	61.5	63.0	68.0	61.0	54.0	46.5	41.3	Il Canonico Butoni.
	Nice	1814—1816	59.60	54.57	−5.50	44.66	50.33	66.80	56.50	37.8	43.2	45.3	47.0	57.0	63.0	66.0	69.0	66.0	60.8	50.0	48.0	Dr. Skirving.
	Naples	1821—1841	61.40	54.58	−6.82	43.66	51.33	66.00	57.33	42.0	43.0	45.3	50.0	58.0	63.0	67.0	68.0	65.0	60.8	47.0	42.5	Professor Piazzini, *Observatory.*
	Naples																	65.0		49.0	46.0	Sig. Boschi, *Obs. Capo di Monte.*
VII.	Leith	1824—1825	48.36	46.90	−2.16	39.40	42.60	55.80	47.0	40.0	39.2	38.2	42.6	47.1	53.6	57.8	56.0	53.6	47.5	40.0	38.9	Brewster,
	Penzance	1807—1820	52.00	50.00	−2.0	52.00	42.60	59.16	50.66	…	42.0	42.0	46.0	53.0	58.0	60.0	59.0	56.0	51.0	45.0	…	Forbes, *Climate of Penzance.*
	Rome	1811—1823	60.70	55.85	−4.85	42.10	54.33	70.66	56.33	41.0	42.3	47.0	54.0	62.0	69.0	72.0	71.0	65.0	55.0	49.0	43.0	Calandrelli, *Collegio Romano.*
VIII.	Leith	1824—1825	48.36	47.02	−1.34	39.47	43.73	57.63	47.66	40.11	39.2	38.9	43.9	48.4	54.9	59.1	58.9	54.9	48.1	40.0	39.1	Brewster,
	London	1817—1819	50.39	48.0	−2.39	39.0	41.0	57.0	54.0	38.0	39.0	40.0	42.0	52.0	59.0	57.0	60.0	56.0	48.0	45.0	36.0	Cay, *Philosoph. Mag.*
	Kinfauns	1813—1818	47.02	44.08	−2.94	34.0	42.33	55.33	44.66	32.0	35.8	38.0	42.0	48.0	54.0	57.0	55.0	51.0	48.0	39.0	34.0	Rev. Mr. Gordon, *Thomson's Annals.*
	Alderley, (Cheshire)	1815—1824	46.80	45.06	−1.74	34.93	43.40	58.00	46.13	34.0	35.8	38.0	42.8	49.4	54.8	59.3	55.9	52.1	45.7	39.4	35.0	Rev. E. Stanley, *Ed. Phil. Journal.*
	Bristol	1803—1808	46.60	46.60	…	43.60	46.00	61.30	47.60	33.20	35.40	35.40	41.2	54.4	59.3	62.4	62.1	57.4	47.0	39.4	35.3	Dr. J. Pole, *London Med. Journal.*
	Chichester	1794—1796	49.50	48.20	−1.30	38.00	46.30	58.80	47.60	35.5	39.0	35.20	41.8	54.4	59.3	62.4	59.3	57.4	49.7	43.0	38.8	Dr. Sandon.
	Gosport	1816—1819	50.24	48.84	−1.40	38.33	46.33	61.0	49.66	39.0	39.0	41.0	46.0	52.0	60.0	62.0	61.0	57.0	49.0	43.0	37.0	Dr. Burney, *Thomson's Annals.*
	Penzance	1807—1820	52.0	…	−1.69	41.33	56.33	74.0	57.0	40.0	44.0	49.0	55.0	65.0	70.0	75.0	77.0	67.0	54.0	50.0	42.0	Forbes.
	Nice	1821—1823	59.60	57.91	…	44.33	56.33	74.0	57.0	43.0	44.0	49.0	55.0	65.0	70.0	75.0	77.0	67.0	54.0	50.0	46.0	Dr. Skirving,
	Idem	1806—1825	59.48	57.30	−2.18	44.83	58.50	70.73	59.16	43.0	46.0	51.0	59.2	65.3	67.5	72.3	72.4	67.5	59.5	50.5	45.5	Dr. Skirving,
	Leghorn	1819—1823	60.0	…	…	44.30	58.50	78.0	…	43.8	44.1	51.0	56.0	65.3	78.0	…	…	…	58.0	57.3	45.2	D. Peebles.
	Florence	1820—1821	59.0	…	…	42.33	56.33	67.40	…	43.0	42.0	48.0	53.0	60.5	62.7	68.0	71.5	64.0	58.0	47.0	43.0	Private Journal.
	Baths of Lucca	1820—1823	55.0	…	−0.20	…	60.30	68.30	62.0	59.0	…	…	53.0	62.0	66.0	67.0	72.0	66.0	63.0	56.0	…	Dr. Todd.
	St. Mich., (Azores)	1825	62.40	62.20	−0.20	59.0	60.30	68.30	62.0	59.0	59.0	60.0	60.0	62.0	66.0	68.0	72.0	66.60	63.0	56.0	56.3	Thomas Blunt, Esq.
IX.	Leith	1824—1825	48.0	47.96	−0.40	39.80	46.30	58.20	48.60	40.3	39.7	39.89	48.0	49.7	56.0	57.0	58.3	56.5	48.8	40.0	39.3	Brewster,
	Dumfermline	1805—1824	45.0	45.02	+0.02	36.10	42.79	55.43	45.75	35.12	37.1	38.7	42.1	48.1	56.0	57.0	55.0	51.1	46.1	49.0	36.1	Rev. H. Fergus, *Ed. Phil. Journal.*
	Bushy Heath	1824—1825	49.82	48.73	−1.09	36.36	45.88	60.36	49.16	37.0	36.6	41.6	46.6	52.3	57.3	63.2	60.6	58.6	47.4	42.9	38.3	Col. Beaufoy, *Annals of Philosophy.*
	Isle of Wight	1809—1818	51.0	50.46	−0.54	39.0	48.66	60.36	51.0	37.0	41.0	44.0	46.0	56.0	62.0	65.0	62.0	58.0	51.0	44.0	39.0	Kirkpatrick, Esq., *Clim. of Penz.*
	Paris	1806—1826	51.50	52.20	+0.70	37.57	52.0	67.20	52.30	36.5	38.8	43.5	52.5	59.2	68.6	65.0	68.0	62.2	51.2	43.5	38.4	M. Bouvard, *Royal Observatory.*
	Pau	1823—1825	54.95	54.95	…	39.35	51.65	65.12	54.93	42.5	41.6	51.7	55.8	58.6	59.9	68.4	67.0	63.8	53.8	47.1	39.6	Mr. Christison, *Private Journal.*
	Pisa	1824	62.88	52.76	−2.19	35.70	…	…	…	42.5	…	51.7	55.8	…	…	…	…	…	…	…	45.0	Private Journal.
XII.	Leith	1824—1825	48.96	48.96	+0.54	40.30	46.50	59.40	49.60	40.8	40.6	42.4	48.0	50.9	57.1	61.0	59.5	57.4	49.9	41.4	39.6	Brewster,
	Clunie, (Perthshire)	1821—1824	47.17	48.89	+1.72	37.20	48.73	61.30	48.36	34.1	37.1	42.4	48.8	55.0	61.1	62.2	60.6	55.5	46.8	42.8	37.2	Rev. — Macritchie, *Ed. Phil. Jour.*
	Kinfauns	1824	47.02	48.29	+1.27	39.93	46.40	59.16	44.70	41.1	40.1	39.7	46.9	58.5	61.1	65.0	58.7	54.8	47.4	41.4	38.6	*Idem.*
	Pisa	1821—1822	60.60	60.60	…	44.0	46.15	72.92	…	43.5	57.0	57.0	67.0	65.9	69.0	72.6	75.0	74.9	60.0	55.0	53.2	Lord Gray,
	Madeira	1826	68.32	68.32	+3.76	62.83	66.15	72.92	71.43	60.8	63.0	65.5	67.0	65.9	69.0	72.6	75.0	74.9	66.0	66.80	64.7	Dr. Heineken, *Phil. Mag.*
X.	Leith	1824—1825	48.36	50.70	+2.34	41.70	48.60	61.20	51.30	42.0	42.2	43.3	49.9	52.5	58.6	63.8	61.2	59.5	51.4	43.0	41.4	Brewster,
	Lausanne	1826	51.50	57.0	+5.50	41.30	56.70	71.13	57.26	38.4	44.2	48.5	53.0	58.5	68.0	72.0	74.0	76.6	57.2	47.5	41.4	Observations for Helvetic Society.
	Paris	1823—1825	54.95	59.36	+4.41	46.05	59.70	71.27	60.41	42.7	44.2	51.6	56.2	65.4	69.2	73.0	72.8	67.0	57.5	54.5	45.9	M. Bouvard, *Royal Observatory.*
	Pau	1806—1825	59.48	67.22	+7.74	55.33	64.40	79.53	69.23	53.5	49.5	55.0	60.3	67.1	66.8	75.3	71.6	69.2	57.5	62.0	56.0	Mr. Christison.
	Nice	1806—1825	60.60	63.09	+2.49	49.66	60.38	77.66	64.89	46.0	52.0	54.4	63.2	70.0	73.0	80.0	83.5	76.7	69.0	62.0	56.0	M. Risso.
	Pisa	1826	60.60	63.09	…	49.66	60.38	77.66	64.89	46.0	52.0	60.2	60.6	75.8	73.0	80.0	80.0	76.0	64.0	54.5	50.7	Mean by three Observers.
	Cadiz	1810—1813	62.88	66.80	+3.92	57.60	64.53	75.03	70.00	55.9	58.6	60.2	64.5	68.9	74.9	80.0	77.5	74.6	71.9	63.5	58.3	Dr. Skirving.

Part	Years	Place	Mean	Higher mean	±	Winter	Spring	Summer	Autumn	Jan	Feb	Mar	Apr	May	Jun	Jul	Aug	Sep	Oct	Nov	Dec	Authority
P.M.	10 years	LONDON	50.39	56.33	+5.94	44.60	55.00	70.46	57.29	41.6	43.5	47.7	54.7	62.5	67.9	71.1	72.9	65.9	58.3	47.6	42.7	Howard, *Higher mean.*
		Environs of London	48.81	56.40	+7.65	42.40	56.60	70.30	56.60	38.3	45.7	48.4	56.0	66.4	68.8	71.8	70.2	65.4	57.0	46.5	42.5	*Idem.*
	1824—1825	Leith	48.36	51.40	+3.04	42.10	49.50	62.10	54.33	38.5	42.7	44.0	50.8	53.6	59.7	64.3	61.9	60.6	52.0	43.7	41.2	Brewster.
	1804—1816	Clifton	52.0	53.33	+1.33	40.66	54.00	68.33	52.76	39.0	40.0	49.0	55.0	58.0	65.0	72.0	68.0	64.0	53.0	46.0	43.0	Dr. Chisholm, (I.P.M.) *Ed. Med. Jour.*
	1815—1824	Alderley	46.80	51.70	+4.90	40.06	51.80	62.26	56.7	39.0	45.0	41.9	52.0	57.6	61.6	68.2	62.8	59.9	56.2	46.1	39.3	Rev. E. Stanley.
	1794—1796	Chichester	49.50	55.20	+5.70	43.0	54.00	66.9	56.66	40.9	45.0	48.4	56.4	59.2	64.0	68.2	68.7	66.5	56.9	47.4	43.1	Dr. Sandon.
	1807—1820	Penzance	52.0	56.0	+4.00	45.66	56.66	67.00	56.33	44.0	48.0	50.0	55.0	62.0	66.0	74.0	67.0	66.5	57.0	53.0	45.0	Dr. Forbes.
	1803—1812	Geneva	49.88	55.83	+5.94	37.83	56.33	72.83	65.10	35.5	46.8	46.8	57.8	66.0	70.5	75.5	74.0	75.5	65.5	46.5	37.5	Pictet.
	1802—1806	Avignon	58.20	65.21	+7.01	47.20	64.16	84.33	65.33	46.8	55.0	58.0	62.2	72.3	83.0	..	85.0	75.0	64.0	54.5	48.0	M. Guerin.
	1821—1826	Nice	59.63	64.74	+5.14	53.33	64.66	75.66	..	51.0	51.2	56.6	65.0	71.0	71.0	..	80.0	75.0	66.1	57.0	54.0	Dr. Skirving.
II.	1814—1816	Pisa	60.60	..	..	48.36	..	..	..	..	52.7	..	..	..	..	..	..	..	65.4	55.4	48.3	Professor Piazzini.
	1821—1822	Idem	60.60	..	..	..	62.63	82.00	66.00	48.0	55.0	55.5	63.4	69.0	80.0	83.0	83.0	78.0	69.0	51.0	49.4	Dr. Todd.
	1810—1823	Leghorn	60.60	65.14	+4.54	52.66	61.66	78.50	..	47.7	49.5	55.0	61.0	69.0	73.0	79.0	79.5	..	65.0	55.0	48.5	Dr. Peebles.
	1820—1823	Baths of Lucca	55.0	63.25	+5.18	49.93	78.00	..	64.50	47.0	49.0	55.5	61.0	69.0	75.0	..	83.5	73.5	61.0	51.0	47.0	Il Canonico Butori.
	1777—1816	Camaiore	58.07	..	..	48.33	61.66	81.50	61.33	49.0	53.0	58.0	62.0	69.0	79.0	83.0	85.0	69.0	64.0	59.0	52.0	Calandrelli.
	1820—1821	Florence	59.0	66.66	+5.96	47.66	64.66	83.33	68.16	52.0	54.0	53.0	62.0	72.0	78.0	88.0	85.0	77.0	68.5	59.0	55.0	Broschi.
	1811—1823	Rome	60.70	67.98	+6.58	59.33	66.66	77.66	70.60	63.0	64.0	58.0	66.0	75.0	76.0	83.0	83.0	80.0	72.0	60.0	55.0	Thomas Blunt, Esq.
	1821—1824	Naples	67.98	69.50	+7.10	63.70	67.00	..	69.66	..	..	65.0	66.0	70.0	76.0	78.0	79.3	76.0	72.0	61.5	64.0	...
	1825	St. Mich.?s (Azores)	62.40	..	..	..	..	..	..	..	..	..	..	..	..	..	..	..	..	..	..	...
III.	1824—1825	Leith	48.36	51.43	+3.07	42.00	49.60	63.20	52.00	42.5	43.7	44.0	51.1	53.6	60.2	64.6	61.9	60.5	51.7	43.7	40.7	Brewster.
	1826	Lausanne	60.60	..	..	51.00	..	..	..	49.0	54.0	54.0	..	..	74.0	76.5	..	74.0	51.0	..	50.0	Observations, &c., Private Journal.
IV.	1824—1825	Leith	48.36	51.16	+2.79	41.60	49.60	62.30	51.20	42.1	42.4	44.0	50.8	54.0	59.8	64.7	62.1	59.9	51.0	42.8	40.5	Brewster.
	1823—1825	Pau	54.95	58.97	+4.02	44.93	58.88	70.70	60.18	42.4	48.5	50.2	59.7	66.6	65.7	75.0	71.4	69.7	56.9	53.8	43.8	Mr. Christison.
Sun Set	1824—1825	Leith	48.36	49.67	+1.31	41.33	47.43	59.33	50.6	42.1	42.8	42.8	48.5	51.0	56.6	61.5	59.9	58.6	50.4	42.8	40.5	Biewster,
	1822—1826	Leghorn	59.60	61.74	+2.14	50.33	60.30	73.33	63.00	44.0	55.0	55.0	55.0	67.0	69.0	74.0	73.0	..	57.0	57.0	52.0	Dr. Skirving,
	1814—1816	Pisa	60.60	..	..	46.33	..	..	..	44.0	53.0	..	..	..	..	..	..	62.7	53.6	46.5	..	Professor Piazzini.
	1821—1822	Pisa	60.60	..	..	..	..	..	..	45.0	5v.5	46.0	..	..	..	..	..	58.0	54.0	..	..	Dr. Todd.
VI.	1810—1812	Cadiz	62.88	66.32	+3.44	57.20	63.66	74.86	69.56	55.9	57.9	59.2	63.7	68.1	72.6	74.8	77.2	71.3	63.2	57.8	..	D. Skirving.
VIII.	1824—1825	Leith	48.36	48.50	+0.14	40.00	46.30	68.90	48.66	40.8	41.3	41.1	46.9	51.0	61.2	61.5	66.6	56.5	48.5	41.0	39.3	Brewster,
	1794—1796	Chichester	49.50	50.90	+0.40	39.60	47.80	62.90	51.60	37.3	41.3	42.8	50.9	55.7	64.1	64.1	61.2	59.9	51.3	43.5	40.2	Dr Sandon.
	1806—1825	Nice	59.20	59.91	+0.71	47.76	56.83	73.10	62.06	45.5	49.0	51.8	55.5	63.2	69.8	74.2	69.8	70.5	62.2	53.5	48.5	M. Risso.
	1825	St. Michael's	62.40	62.60	+0.20	57.60	62.00	68.30	62.30	59.0	50.0	60.0	62.0	64.0	69.8	68.0	69.0	63.0	54.0	36.5	55.0	Thomas Blunt, Esq.
IX.	1824—1825	Leith	48.36	47.40	−0.64	39.90	45.20	57.66	48.30	40.7	39.9	43.0	45.7	49.5	55.3	55.7	57.6	55.7	48.4	41.0	39.2	Brewster,
	1821—1823	Leghorn	60.60	59.45	−1.30	44.40	47.20	71.80	61.66	45.0	43.2	50.0	56.3	75.0	..	..	..	69.0	52.0	54.0	36.0	Dr. Peebles.
	1811—1823	Rome	60.60	..	..	47.33	57.00	..	..	46.0	44.0	51.0	56.0	64.0	69.0	73.4	73.0	69.0	62.0	54.0	38.0	Calendrelli.
X.	1824—1825	Leith	48.36	47.40	−0.96	39.88	44.60	57.40	47.80	40.7	39.9	39.8	45.0	56.9	56.7	58.5	55.1	55.7	48.0	40.3	39.2	Brewster
	1821—1824	Clumie	47.17	45.45	−1.72	37.33	47.29	52.96	44.33	37.3	37.8	37.8	46.4	52.7	53.2	53.0	47.9	52.0	44.1	41.0	39.9	Rev. — Macritchie.
	1824	Kinfauns	47.02	45.63	−1.39	39.60	42.66	54.43	45.83	41.3	39.5	37.5	47.2	53.5	54.2	56.4	52.0	45.3	44.5	40.2	36.0	Lord Gray.
	1815—1824	Alderley	46.80	44.80	−2.00	35.70	42.72	54.60	45.83	34.8	36.2	38.6	47.9	53.5	54.8	55.5	51.8	51.8	54.5	51.0	36.1	Rev. E. Stanley.
	1821—1822	Pisa	60.60	..	..	43.50	..	..	..	38.5	44.0	50.0	..	..	..	..	..	55.5	51.0	48.0	..	Dr. Todd.
XI.	1824—1825	Leith	48.36	46.70	−1.66	39.73	43.30	55.80	47.43	40.6	39.5	39.4	45.7	48.1	53.7	57.7	56.0	54.7	47.7	39.9	39.0	Brewster,
	1824	Pisa	60.60	..	..	40.00	..	..	..	38.0	43.0	43.0	49.0	49.0	..	..	..	..	55.5	44.0	41.0	Plain of Pisa, 6 miles S.S.E. of Town.

TABLE VII.—Showing the range of the barometer for each month and for the whole year.

NAMES OF THE PLACES.	Annual Mean Temperature.	Annual Mean height of Barometer	Range for the whole Year.	Jan.	Feb.	March	April.	May.	June.	July.	August	Sept.	Oct.	Nov.	Dec.	NAMES OF OBSERVERS, PERIODS OF OBSERVATION, &c.
LONDON	50.39	*29.895	1.998	1.429	1.350	1.299	1.070	0.914	0.830	0.691	0.759	0.898	1.158	1.458	1.450	Howard, 1806—1816.
Idem	.....	.....	.....	1.600	1.360	1.260	1.110	1.090	0.640	0.790	0.730	0.860	1.380	0.920	1.130	Daniell, 1819—1823.
Edinburgh	47.31	*29.624	.....	1.850	1.700	1.000	0.950	0.900	0.600	0.850	1.250	1.300	1.400	1.150	1.500	Medical Observations, 1734-5.
County of Antrim	47.87	29.530	.....	1.400	1.400	1.700	1.100	0.900	0.800	0.700	0.700	1.300	1.200	1.100	1.600	Edinburgh Medical Journal.
Kendal	48.03	29.530	2.060	1.190	1.510	1.630	0.710	0.840	0.870	0.760	1.080	1.060	1.260	0.960	1.890	S. Marshall, Esq., 1827: *Phil. Mag.*
Alderley, Cheshire	46.80	29.460	1.700	1.683	1.355	1.410	1.200	0.965	0.867	0.787	0.875	0.974	1.230	1.395	1.575	Rev. E. Stanley, 1815—1824.
Cheltenham	51.32	29.627	1.550	1.150	0.910	1.100	1.080	0.630	0.590	0.550	0.810	0.900	1.060	1.210	1.000	Moss, 1825-26.
Gosport	50.24	29.900	1.790	0.970	0.950	1.510	0.840	1.050	0.690	0.700	1.030	0.840	1.290	1.120	1.510	Dr. Burney, 1827.
Sidmouth	52.10	29.964	.....	1.410	0.990	1.310	1.000	0.850	0.780	0.790	0.710	0.800	1.240	1.140	1.390	Dr. Clarke, 1812—1814.
Penzance	52.16	29.620	1.950	1.360	1.070	1.080	0.940	0.600	0.570	0.763	0.680	0.990	0.940	0.940	1.140	Dr. Forbes, 1818-19.
Nantes	55.62	*29.830	1.817	1.172	1.376	1.021	1.419	1.110	0.843	0.688	0.532	0.795	1.332	0.706	1.065	Huette, 1824-5.
Montpelier	57.60	29.747	.....	0.917	0.854	0.751	0.588	0.464	0.676	0.464	0.397	0.532	0.706	0.843	0.917	M. Mejan.
Milan	55.80	29.579	1.279	0.961	0.958	0.871	0.788	0.614	0.439	0.437	0.435	0.436	0.614	0.871	0.958	L'Abbate Cesaris, 1763—1817.
Genoa	.....	.....	.....	0.706	1.065	0.917	0.532	0.444	0.353	0.588	0.444	0.588	0.588	.....	.....	J. Fratelli Mojon, 1802.
Florence	59.00	29.884	1.508	1.065	0.977	0.588	0.799	0.588	0.397	0.400	0.464	0.731	1.332	0.706	1.065	Ximenian Observatory.
Rome	60.70	29.893	1.221	0.843	0.854	0.977	0.676	0.588	0.442	0.397	0.360	0.532	0.676	0.751	0.917	Calendrelli, 1811—1823.
Naples	61.40	29.554	1.154	0.888	0.843	0.888	0.710	0.355	0.552	0.266	0.355	0.488	0.552	0.621	0.621	Broschi, 1821—1824.
Madeira	64.56	*30.030	1.211	0.618	0.657	0.659	0.482	0.500	0.258	0.373	0.260	0.311	0.497	1.010	0.700	Heineken, 1826.

* The asterisk marks where correction is made for the expansion of the mercury by the heat.

TABLE VIII.—SHOWING THE MEAN QUANTITIES OF RAIN, IN INCHES AND PARTS OF INCHES, FOR EACH MONTH AND FOR THE WHOLE YEAR.

Columns Jan.–Dec. fall under the heading **MEAN MONTHLY QUANTITIES OF RAIN.**

NAMES OF THE PLACES	Mean Annual Temperature	Mean Annual Quantity of Rain	Ratio of the Mean Annual Temperature to the Annual Quantity of Rain	Average number of Days on which rain falls	Jan.	Feb.	March	April	May	June	July	Aug.	Sept.	Oct.	Nov.	Dec.	NAMES OF OBSERVERS, PERIODS OF OBSERVATION, &c.
LONDON	50.39	*20.686	2.4350	178	1.464	1.250	1.172	1.279	1.636	1.738	2.448	1.807	1.842	2.092	2.222	1.736	Dalton, 40 years.
Idem		24.804	2.0315	178	1.959	1.482	1.299	1.692	1.822	1.920	2.637	2.125	1.921	2.522	2.998	2.427	Howard, 20 years.
Edinburgh	47.31	23.500	2.0631		1.090	1.360	0.880	0.990	1.940	2.030	0.860	1.690	2.230	3.460	4.140	2.890	Adie, 1824, 1825.
Kinfauns	47.02	24.060	1.9542	137	1.400	1.300	1.120	1.700	1.500	2.250	1.050	1.850	2.270	3.070	3.600	3.050	Lord Gray, 1824, 1825.
Glasgow		21.331			1.595	1.741	1.184	0.979	1.641	1.343	2.303	2.746	1.617	2.297	1.904	1.981	Dalton, 17 years.
Dumfries		36.919			3.095	2.837	2.164	2.017	2.568	2.974	3.236	3.199	4.350	4.143	3.174	3.142	Idem, 16 years.
Kendal	46.22	53.944	0.8565	176	5.299	5.126	3.151	2.996	3.490	2.722	4.959	5.039	4.874	5.439	4.785	6.064	Dalton, 25 years.
Alderney (Cheshire)	46.80	32.889	1.4230	188	1.786	2.125	2.843	2.096	2.559	2.742	3.468	3.153	2.565	3.125	3.205	3.238	Rev. E. Stanley, 1815—1821.
Lancaster		39.714			3.461	2.995	1.753	2.180	2.460	2.512	4.140	4.561	3.751	4.151	3.775	3.955	Dalton, 20 years.
Liverpool		34.118			2.177	1.847	1.523	2.104	2.573	2.816	3.663	3.311	3.654	3.724	3.441	3.288	Idem, 18 years.
Manchester		36.140			2.310	2.568	2.098	2.010	2.895	2.502	3.697	3.665	3.281	3.922	3.360	3.832	Idem, 33 years.
Chatsworth		27.664			2.196	1.632	1.322	2.078	2.118	2.286	3.006	2.435	2.289	3.079	2.634	2.569	Idem, 16 years.
New Malton	47.65	36.740	1.2864	137	1.160	1.220	2.830	2.110	2.270	2.720	1.170	2.850	5.610	6.250	4.380	4.170	Mr. Stockton, 1824. (Phil. Mag.)
Bushey Park	49.82	30.596	1.5344		0.849	3.694	1.364	2.133	3.710	3.270	1.729	2.433	3.260	2.862	2.546	2.746	Colonel Beaufoy, 1824, 1825.
Bristol		31.000															Dr. Cole.
Gosport	50.24	29.965	1.6900	135	1.000	0.820	3.145	1.910	2.125	1.660	1.115	2.060	3.835	4.635	1.835	5.625	Dr. Burney, 1827.
Sidmouth	52.10	27.290	1.9095	195	3.850	2.340	0.500	2.500	1.670	2.030	2.280	1.180	1.750	3.500	1.990	2.700	Dr. Clarke, 1813, 1814.
Helston	50.94	44.964	1.1508	170	4.177	3.770	3.320	2.087	2.685	3.330	2.987	4.140	3.669	4.750	4.512	4.887	Mr. Moyle, 1823, 1824.
Penzance	52.16	44.412	1.1740		3.546	3.257	3.876	1.819	3.064	2.145	2.963	3.496	3.437	5.613	5.186	6.010	Mr. E. Giddy, 1821, 1827.
Paris	51.00	*18.694	2.7347		1.228	1.232	1.190	1.185	1.767	1.697	1.800	1.900	1.550	1.780	1.720	1.600	Dalton, 15 years.
Toulouse	52.50	25.120	2.0900	82													Poitevin, 1796, 1805.
Montpelier	57.60	29.898	1.9265	55	2.131	1.621	3.730	2.664	2.664	1.250	0.399	0.666	1.621	3.375	4.999	4.841	Blanpain, 10 years.
Marseilles	59.50	*15.610	3.2718		1.705	0.756	0.852	0.650	0.959	0.756	1.705	0.959	1.833	2.558	1.598	1.270	Burel, 33 years.
Toulon	59.90	19.712	3.0887		2.131	1.065	1.332	1.598	1.598	0.621	0.355	0.621	2.576	2.753	2.664	2.398	
Turin	53.50	32.898	1.6000		1.508	0.581	2.079	4.319	4.189	4.492	3.592	2.727	2.639	3.408	2.116	1.248	Vassali Eandi, 1803—1818.
Milan	55.80	37.838	1.4700	103	2.842	2.024	2.306	3.090	3.730	3.197	2.839	3.016	3.197	4.156	4.351	3.090	Cesaris, 1763—1807.
Florence	59.00	*31.687	1.8556	117	3.581	0.991	3.273	2.036	3.485	1.961	1.151	0.660	2.515	3.273	3.678	5.083	Ximinian Observatory, 1824, 1825.
Rome	60.70	*31.173	1.9471		4.263	1.687	2.043	1.776	2.486	1.687	1.243	1.243	2.309	5.507	3.375	3.553	Calendrelli, 1811—1823.
Madeira	64.56	25.096	2.5600	73	3.217	1.757	1.510	1.520	1.072	0.347	0.372	0.405	1.067	2.082	8.577	3.100	Dr. Heineken, 1825, 1826, 1827.

* The Asterisk denotes those places where the rain-gauge stood at a considerable height above the ground.

TABLE IX.—SHOWING THE RELATIVE PREVALENCE OF DIFFERENT KINDS OF WEATHER FOR EACH MONTH, AND FOR THE WHOLE YEAR.

NUMBER OF DAYS DURING WHICH THE DIFFERENT KINDS OF WEATHER HAVE PREVAILED IN EACH MONTH.

NAMES OF THE PLACES.	Number of days on which each particular kind of weather prevails, during the year.			January.			February.			March.			April.			May.			June.			July.			August.			September.			October.			November.			December.			NAMES OF OBSERVERS, PERIODS OF OBSERVATION, &c.
	Fine	Cloudy or Variable.	Days on which any Rain falls.	Fine	Cloudy or Variable	Rain falls	Fine	Cloudy or Variable	Rain falls	Fine	Cloudy or Variable	Rain falls	Fine	Cloudy or Variable	Rain falls	Fine	Cloudy or Variable	Rain falls	Fine	Cloudy or Variable	Rain falls	Fine	Cloudy or Variable	Rain falls	Fine	Cloudy or Variable	Rain falls	Fine	Cloudy or Variable	Rain falls	Fine	Cloudy or Variable	Rain falls	Fine	Cloudy or Variable	Rain falls	Fine	Cloudy or Variable	Rain falls	
LONDON	218		178			14		4	16		4	13		1	14			16		1	12			16			16			12			16			15			18	Howard, 1807—1816.
Kinfauns	156	54	147			8			10			11			9			10			9			7			12			6			18			11			17	Lord Gray, 1824—1825.
County of Antrim			155	15	2	14		4	14	13	4	14		1	17			6	17	1	12	11	4	16		7	20		1	6	10	9	12	7	11	12	9	10	12	Edinburgh Medical Journal.
Cork	228		157			6			6			13			11	11		11			10			5			11			12			16			20			16	
New Malton, Yorks.	177		137	10	6	14	10	6	15		3	18		10	14		7	16	14	3	14		5	17		3	11		4	15		7	17	14	5	16			15	Mr. Stockton, 1823, 1824.
Alderly, Cheshire	156	60	188	14	7	15	13	6	15	16	3	13	19	1	10	16	7	9	17		12	17	5	13	21	1	16	20	2	8	13	1	17	13	5	16	11	7	11	Rev. E. Stanley.
Clifton	196	34	149	14		10	12		13	18		12	20		10	17		12	20		11	19		14	18		13	15		12	16		16	14		17	9	3	18	Dr. Chisholme, 1814, 1815.
Sidmouth	170		135	17		17	13		14	18		13	15		10	18		14	18		10	20		12	18		13	18		12	15		15	13		17	13		18	Dr. Clarke, 1819—1814.
Helston, Cornwall	119	91	195	14	6	16	9	11	20	10	10	13	10	8	10	12	9	13	11	10	11	18	6	12	15	7	13	15	8	11	19	10	15	14	14	17		15	18	Mr. Moyle, 1823, 1824.
Penzance	114	87	155	14	7	16	8	5	15	17	4	13	15		7	14		10	10	7	5	13	5	8	13		9	12		12	15		11	13		12	4		12	Forbes, 1807—1820.
Idem	144	115	164	16	12	7			8	10	10	10	8	8	10	13	9	13	18	7	11	20	6	8	18	7	6	16	8	7	11	10	11	14	14	9	9	15	12	Mr. E. C. Gieldy, 21 years.
Nantes	155	101	106	12	13	7		9	5	17	4	11	9		9	10	10	10	8	9	7	18	6	3	15	12	3	15	7	9	14	5	12	17	4	8	4	12	10	Huette, 1824, 1825.
Pau	155		109	13	10	10	10	9	12	9	4	11	7		7	7		7		7	6	18	6	8	12	7	6	14	9	9	12	5	12			12			10	Mr. Christison, 1829—1824.
Toulouse			113		5	8		4	5		9	6		11	7	11	11	7	16	10	4	20	9	2	15	11	3	12	10	5	9	8	6		7	8			11	
Montpelier	180	130	80	9	5	8	15	6	7	13	9	9	15	11	7	13	9	9	16	5	9	21	4	6	21	4	5	12	5	8	9	6	7	9	7	14	8	7	8	Poitevrain, 1796—1806.
Marseilles			55					1									4	4		5							11	5		13	6	6		7	9	12			8	Thulis and Blanpain.
Genoa	166	75	123	9	5	17	15	6	15	13	9	13	15	11	4	13	11	9	16	10	14	20	9	5	15	11	5	12	10	8	9	12	14	9	7	14	10	7	14	J. Fratelli Mojon.
Camajore	164	98	103	19	2	12	12	8	10	10	10	3	14	4	12	15	7	9	11	5	15	21	4	6	7	6	7	12	7	8	12	13	12	14	12	8	9	13	9	Il Canonico Butori, 1777—1816.
Florence				13	5	13	14	5	9	15	6	11	15	6	9	17	5	10	18	5	7	23	3	5	23	3	5	18	4	8	15	2	14	14	4	6	13	5	13	Ximenian Observatory, 1825.
Pisa	197	51	117	17	3	11	17	5	9	13	8	10	17	6	8	18	7	6	17	4	9	29	1	1	16	3	12	17	5	8	17	3	11	18	6	6	15	5	11	Piazzini, 1815—1817.
Rome	210	58	97																																				Calandrelli, 1811—1823.
Naples																																							Broschi, 1821—1824.
Madeira	201	91	73	10	6	15	21	7		17	6	9	17	7	2	17	6	8	12	17	1	20	8	3	23	8		9	10	11	19	5	7	10	3	17	12	13	6	Heineken, 1826.

TABLE X.—Showing the Number of Patients received annually into the Hospital of the Santo Spirito, at Rome, with the Population of the City, for twenty-five years.

Years.	Population of Rome.	Number of Patients received into the S. Spirito Hospital.
1801	146,384	8,891
1802	144,212	12,586*
1803	140,003	17,714*
1804	136,762	8,881
1805	134,973	7,239
1806	134,973	8,330
1807	136,356	5,599
1808	136,854	5,972
1809	136,268	6,416
1810	123,023	8,892
1811	128,850	11,880
1812	121,608	9,791
1813	117,882	5,651
1814	120,505	6,072
1815	128,384	7,631
1816	128,997	7,505
1817	131,356	15,709*
1818	133,812	16,236*
1819	134,161	11,892
1820	135,046	10,572
1821	135,171	12,981
1822	136,085	10,180
1823	136,269	8,074
1824	138,510	8,075
1825	138,730	6,401

TABLE XI.— Showing the Number of Sick received during the different Months of 1812. The Increase during July, August, and September is entirely owing to the Malaria Fevers, which occur chiefly during these Months. I have selected 1812 because the Reports of that year are very complete.

January . . .   857

February . .   609

March . . .   522

April   460

May   384

June   325

July 1,004

August . . . 1,837

September . 1,267

October . . .   818

November . .   633

December . .   600

* The great increase in the number of sick in 1802 and 1803, and again in 1817 and 1818, was owing to a petechial fever which prevailed in Italy during these two periods.

NOTES TO TABLES OF CLIMATE.

1. London. (A.) Howard; from the observations made at the
apartments of the Royal Society, Somerset
House, 1797—1816 : 1787—1816, 50°.456.
Climate of London. Mean of maxima and
minima, 1820—1822, 49°.30. Daniell, *Essay
on the Climate of London.* Range of mean
annual temperature during 30 years, 4°.8.
Howard.

(B.) Deduced from the average extremes; 1820
—1823. Daniell. Maximum temperature,
during 30 years, 96° 13th July, 1808. Minimum during the same period—5°. 9th
February, 1816. Howard.

(C.) Average difference of the higher and lower
mean, 1797—1806. Howard. Mean daily
range according to Daniell, 13°.6; mean
maximum, 56°.1 ; mean minimum, 42°.5.

(D.) Mean difference of the temperature of the
same hours of successive days; calculated
from Daniell's Meteorological Journal, 1820
—1823.

2. Edinburgh. (A.) A. Adie, Esq.; 10 A. M., 10 P. M., 1824,
1825; at Canaan Cottage, 1½ mile south of
Edinburgh Castle, 3 miles from the sea, and
260 feet above its level. *Edinburgh Journal
of Science.* Mean of year 47°.8; Winter,
38°.6, Spring, 46°.4, Summer, 58°.2, Autumn, 48°.4,—warmest month, 59°.4, coldest
month, 58°.3. Playfair.

   (B.) Adie, *ut supra.*

3. Leith. (A.) Dr. Brewster; from the valuable observations
made at Leith Fort, 1824, 1825.

   (B.) "The measure of the daily change of temperature." Brewster. *Edin. Journ. of Science.*

4. Kinfauns Castle. (A.) Lord Gray; 10 A. M., 10 P. M., 140
feet above the level of the sea; 1825,
48°.319; mean of maxima and minima
49°.048. *Edinburgh Philosophical Journal,*
XXIV. XXVIII.

5. Dublin. Kirwan.

6. County of Antrim, Northern coast of; 1814. *Edinburgh
Medical Journal.*

7. Kendal. Dalton.

8. Alderley Rectory, (near Knutsford, Cheshire.) (A.) The
Rev. E. Stanley; 1815, 1824, mean of 8
A. M., 2 P. M., and 10 P. M., corrected for
each month by Dr. Brewster's table, as
deduced from the Leith Fort observations.

   (B.) Average of extremes of 10 years. Extreme
range in 10 years, 84°—1°=83.

   (C.) Mean difference of 8 A. M. and 2 P. M. *Edin.
Philosophical Journal,* XXIV.

9. New Malton. Yorkshire. Mr. Stockton; 1823, 1824; 92
feet above the level of the sea. *Annals of
Philosophy.*

10. Oxford.   Dr. Robertson, Radcliffe Observatory; 1816—

1821; mean of maxima and minima.
Edinburgh Philosophical Journal.

11. Environs of London, viz., Plaistow, Stratford, and Tottenham. Howard, *ut supra.*

    (A.) 1807—1816. Mean of maxima and minima.

    (B.) Average extremes, 1807—1816.

    (C.) Average difference of the higher and lower mean, 1807—1816.

12. Bushey Heath. Colonel Beaufoy; 1824—1825. Mean of extremes. *Annals of Philosophy.*

12. (A.) Chichester. Dr. Sandon; 1794—1796. Mean of 8 A. M., and 8 P. M.; cross of Chichester 32 feet above the level of the sea.

13. Chiswick. Garden of the Horticultural Society, 1826. *Transactions of the Horticultural Society.*

14. Gosport. Dr. Burney; corrected for each month by Brewster's table, *ut supra.*

15. Isle of Wight, — Kirkpatrick, Esq.; 9 A. M., 1809—1818, Forbes, *Climate of Penzance.*

16. Cheltenham. Moss; 1821, 1825, 1826; mean of extremes. Thomas, *Practical Observations,* &c.

17. Sidmouth. Dr. Clarke; 1812—1814; mean of 9 A. M., and 2 P. M. *Edinburgh Medical Journal.*

18. Helston, Cornwall. Mr. Moyle; 1823, 1824; 105 feet above the level of the sea. *Edinburgh Med. Journal.*

19. Penzance. Mr. E. C. Giddy; (A.) 1821—1827; mean of maxima and minima; mean of 8 A. M., and 2 P. M., 1807—1827, as follows, January, 43°.0, February, 45°.5, March, 47°.0, April, 51°.7, May, 58°.5, June, 62°.5, July. 65°.5 August, 64°.5, September, 60°.0, October, 55°.5, November, 49°.0, December, 46°.0. These, corrected by Brewster's table for the difference of temperature of the hours

of observation, and the temperature of all
the twenty-four hours, would give January
41°.80, February, 44°.30, March, 45°.80,
April, 49°.80, May, 56°.80, June, 61°.80,
July, 63°.80, August, 62°.80, September,
58°.30, October, 53°.70, November, 47°.0,
December, 44°.10; Winter, 43°.40, Spring,
50°.80, Summer, 62°.80, Autumn, 53°.00;
annual mean 52.50, nearly corresponding
with the mean of the extremes.

(B.) Average extremes, 1821—1827. Extreme
range during 21 years, 84°—19°=65°.

(C.) Mean difference of 7 A. M., and 2 P. M.

(D.) Forbes ; *Climate of Penzance.*

20. Geneva. (A.) Pictet, mean of sunrise and 2 P. M.; 1080
feet above the level of the sea. Saussure,
50°.74; Berne, 49°.30: difference of warmest and coldest month, 36°.12. Zurich, 47°.8,
difference of warmest and coldest month,
31°.10.

(B.) Difference of the mean of sunrise and of 2
P. M. Annual range at Sion, 92°—9=83°.
1819, 92°.—2°=94°.

21 Paris. (A.) Royal Observatory; mean of extremes; M.
Boward, 1806—1826.

(B.) Mean difference of sunrise and 3 P. M.

(C.) Calculated by Dr. H. C. Lombard, of
Geneva.

22. Nantes. Huette, Observatory; 46 metres above the level of
the sea, and 25 from the ground; 1824,
1825, 55°.94. Duplessis and Bondin.

23. Bourdeaux. Humboldt from Guyot.

24. Pau. (A.) Mr. Christison; at Chateau Billère, from September 1822 to July 1824; and at Pau, Hotel
de Place, from July 1824 to May 1825.

(B.) Mean difference of 9 A. M., and noon annual
of range at Toulouse, 81°—24=57°.

(c.) Mean difference at 9 A. M., 12 A. M., and
4 P. M.

25. Montpelier. Poitevin; 1796—1806. *Sur le Climat de
Montpelier.* 58° mean of 12 years; Mejan.
Nismes, 60°.26.

26 Avignon. (A.) M. Guerin; Musée Calvet; about 70 feet
above the level of the sea; sunrise and
2 P. M.

(B.) Mean difference of sunrise and 2 P. M. Extreme range in 12 years, 101°—12°=89°.

27 Marseilles. (A.) Thulis and Blanpain, Royal Observatory;
about 160 feet above the level of the sea;
1806—1815. *Statistique des Bouches du
Rhone.* 60°.10. St. Jaque de Sylvabelle.
Aix 56°.66; 309 feet above the level of the
sea.

(B.) Range at Marseilles 93°—20°=73°; at Aix
102°—19°=83°.

28 Toulon. M. Burel, Naval Hospital; 1749—1781.
Statistique des Bouches du Rhone.

29 Nice. (A.) M. Risso; 1806—1825; mean of 8 A. M.
and of 8 P.M., corrected by Brewster's table.
Histoire Naturelle de l'Europe Meridionale.
Dr. Skirving, November, 1820, to February, 1826; mean of sunrise and 2 P. M.
Both these series of observations nearly co-
incide.

(B.) Dr. Skirving; mean difference of sunrise and
2 P.M.

(c.) Idem; the mean difference of successive
days at sun-rise and at 2 P. M.

30 Genoa. I. Fratelli Majon. Humboldt, 60°.26.

31. Baths of Lucca. Dr. Todd.

32 Camajore.   State of Lucca at the foot of the Appenines, 105 feet above the level of the sea.

       (A.) Il Canonico Butori; 1777—1816.   Lucca 60°.44 ; 40 feet above the level of the sea.

       (B.) Range 88°.50 —24°.00 = 64°.50; extreme range in 40 years 99°—18°=81°.

33 Sienna.   At Belvidera; 1786—1791 ; furnished by Professor Grotanelli.

34 Florence.   Ximenian Observatory, Scuole Pie; 205 feet above the level of the sea; mean of three daily observations; 1824—1825. Temperature within doors 61°.50, out of doors 58°.75. Humboldt 61°.52. Bologna 56°.30. Verona 55°.76. Venice 56°.48. Padua 56°.30.

35 Leghorn.   (A.) Dr. Peebles and others.

       (B.) Mean difference of 8 A. M. and 2 P. M.

36 Pisa.   Deduced from several Journals. 60°.0. Piazzini.

37 Rome.   (A.) Observatory of the Roman College, 163 feet above the level of the Mediterranean and 101 feet from the level of the ground ; 1811 —1823. The mean of the evening observation at 9 P. M. has been preferred to the mean of 7 A. M. and 2 P. M. *Effemeride Astronomiche.* 60°.08. Calandrelli. 63°.44. W. Humboldt.

       (*) It freezes on an average about ten times in every year, and snow falls about twice a year.

       (B.) Mean difference of 7 A. M. and 2 P. M. Extreme range during 13 years 101°—22°=89°.

       c.) Mean difference of successive days at 7 A.M., 2 P. M., and at 9 P. M.

38 Naples.   (A.) Broschi, Observatory at Capo di Monte ; 148 metres above the level of the sea ;

mean of sunrise and 2 P. M.; 1821—1824.
Toaldo, 63°.5. Palermo, 63°.60. Scena,
Topografia di Palermo.

(B.) Mean difference of sunrise and 2 P. M. Extreme range during 5 years 95°—26°=69°.

(c.) Mean difference of successive days at sunrise and 2 P. M.

38 Bis.   Mr. William Black; *Edinburgh Philosophical Journal, September,* 1821. Mean of 3 years, affording a view of what temperature a person might be exposed to sailing indiscriminately in different parts of the Mediterranean.

39 Cadiz.   (A.) Dr. Skirving; September 1810 to August 1812, on board ship in Cadiz Bay, at noon and 6 P. M., corrected by Brewster's table; Madrid 59°.0; 2040 feet above the level of the sea. Lisbon 62°. Balbi. *Essai statistique sur le Portugal.*

(B.) Calculated by Dr. C. Lombard.

39 St. Michaels. (c.) Thomas Blunt, Esq., 1825—Mean of 8 A. M. and 8 P. M.

40 Madeira   (A.) Dr. Heineken, *Funchal;* 1826. Mean deduced from mean maxima and mean minima. Gourlay; mean of extremes; 1793—1802; mean annual temperature, 66°.21. Winter, 62°.53, Spring, 63°.00, Summer, 70°.50, Autumn, 69°.20; January, 61°.40, February, 62°.20, March, 61°.30, April, 62°.10, May, 65°.60, June, 67°.40, July, 71°.10, August, 72°.90, September, 72°.80, October, 69°.20, November, 65°.60, December, 63°.00. Heberden 67°.30; mean annual temperature, as corrected by M. Schouw.

(B.) † Gourlay, average of 18 years. (?) Heineken 1826.

(c.) Mean difference of maxima and minima.

(D.) Mean difference of successive days at 10 A. M., and 10 P. M.

41 Santa Cruz, Isle of Teneriffe, Von Buch, from the Journal of Don Francisco Escolar; mean of sunrise and of noon.

42 Cairo.   Humboldt, from Nouet.

GAULTER, Printer, 5, Lovell's Court, Paternoster Row.

Milton Keynes UK
Ingram Content Group UK Ltd.
UKHW032319161024
449665UK00001B/43